CW00411563

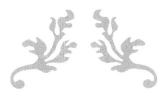

SENDA

By Emeel Safie

The movement is the measure of the universe

Emeel Safie

Introduction

"Senda" is a Spanish word meaning "the path".

Between birth and death, we all experience pain, but in the end we will all die. There are different levels of pain on this path, and it is our choice how long we live suffering at each level, accepting the pain and learning from it.

Your pain may come from the mind put in the box, from the way you move the body, how you deal with people, how you plan your time, the weather, malnutrition, etc. It signals that there is a problem and calls for solving it. The pain is not an enemy, it is a challenge!

Pain!

When I look around I see:

Someone having pain in the neck or lower back when lying down

Someone having pain in the neck and shoulders while sitting

Pain in the knee and hip when standing up

Someone having pain in the ankles, knees, hips and lower back when walking

Or pain in the shoulders, neck, lower back and hip because of wearing the backpack

And a lot of injuries from doing sports.

Why is it normal for those who have

- thyroid disease or are deaf to not have flexible jaws?

- Alzheimer or migraine to not have a flexible neck?

- heart, lungs or seasonal allergy problems to not have flexible shoulders?

- infertility, genital problems or digestive system problems to not have flexible hips?

And I also do not understand why it is Normal to be:

- a dancer and have pain in the knees, hips, lower back or ankles!

- a golfer and tennis player with pain in the elbow and wrist!

- a runner or soccer player with pain in the knees, hips or back!

- a swimmer with pain in the shoulders!

- a professional sportsman and stop your career or give up on your dream just because of an injury!

5

What is Pain?

Pain is the language between the body and you that is there to protect you and warn you when the body is getting damaged.

Why do we get pain?

When you keep moving and doing things all your day in a repetitive way, the body starts to warn you by giving you pain in the parts that you are using.

How about starting to avoid getting pain?

To balance something, you have to know first what is the Zero position of this something. Then you need to start doing the opposite (relative to the Zero) of what you did earlier, and after that you can start moving and doing your things differently.

Senda was born from this question

What if we think about it differently?!

Your balanced mind makes your moves balanced and your balanced moves make your mind balanced.

The mind is like a sponge: the more you see, observe and learn, the more you have to squeeze out to keep the most important information to yourself. The rest can be thrown away so that tomorrow you are able to take in the new information again.

When you have a mental issue with yourself or with someone else, try this technique: Ask a logical question in the 'wrong' moment. This will let the emotions drop down and the brain will take over.

Examples:

a. When you have a mental issue with yourself, ask yourself: Why do I not enjoy the nice moments for as long as the bad ones? Did I move before my breakfast? Where did I go yesterday?

b. When you have mental issues with someone else, ask this someone: Did you buy tomatoes and bananas? Did you drink water before or after the food yesterday? What did you read yesterday?

Thinking differently about everything keeps your mind flexible and that gives you the ability to adapt very quickly to any situation in this life.

Examples:

a) If you have a hard time with your family, stop treating them the way you do, and imagine you are a stranger. How would this stranger react to the situation in your family?

b) If you find yourself getting too involved into arguing with someone, just stop it and gently change the topic. Think about how to later tell them what is bothering you in a different way.

c) If you have problems studying or not achieving your goals, stop pursuing them for a while. Do something else, listen to someone who has pain. Then think about how you could achieve your goals using the least amount of energy and time.

d) If you are not satisfied with your job, start reducing the working hours and do the things you love to do, work/train very hard on these things. When you are ready, quit your job and find another that utilizes the things you trained – or maybe start your own business.

Senda is the detail in each movement, it is not a sport art, it is a lifestyle – it is happening before, during and after the movement. This is because it is very important to enter, make and leave the movement with full awareness.

That is why, you walk along the Senda path when you are shopping, driving, walking to the bus and while sitting in a waiting room, but also when you are training. You are aware of each detail in how you sit, how you stand, how you walk, etc.

The treasure of our beautiful mechanism

Our body is an amazingly beautiful mechanism, but because we live inside of it, we do not always appreciate this treasure. Unfortunately, it often takes an illness – your own or of somebody close to you – to make you see all the value that your body is creating for you. We just get one body in this life, so why not to treat it in a luxurious way?

Back in 2007, the vision and concept of Senda came to my life when I realized that personal beliefs and principles often do not fit one's body.

Guided by the idea of saving time and energy, I started collecting information necessary for improving the way how people move –and, eventually, how they live. This improvement is achieved by focusing on the joints, by doing the exact opposite of any movement carrying weight, and by moving differently.

When you move any part of your body in any particular, repetitive way all the time, it wears out and becomes vulnerable. To keep it healthy and functional in the long run, you need to find the exact opposites of movements (the counterparts, the complementing moves) for each movement you make. The opposite can be found by simplifying the movement as many examples in this book illustrate. Doing the exact opposite movement neutralizes negative effects of any movement. Keep in mind that also the new movements – with which you improve yourself – need to be neutralized.

The unbalanced positions of your joints cause damage to your muscles while you are awake. During your sleep, your body tries to fix this damage by involuntarily contracting and stretching these muscles. For example, when you are sitting still, your abs (abdominals) are contracted and your lower back muscles are stretched or overstretched. In your sleep, then, the body activates its self-defense mechanism, contracting lower back muscles and stretching the abs. Doing Senda will give your body the balance it needs while you are still awake so that it will not have to use its self-defense for correcting the unbalanced positions in the sleep anymore.

What this book is about

This book is not just about movement. It also is about how to change your lifestyle to make your life movely livly (move and live subconsciously), more enjoyable.

The book is devoted to the style that we call "Senda", invented and developed by me from my rich experience of the last decade as a dance, pilates, yoga, martial arts, athletics and fitness trainer, and from experiences shared by my father Mohammad Safie as well as other sports professionals and amateurs. I also collected relevant experience from various types of massage therapy: Feet and Hands Reflexology, Ayurveda, Abhyanga, Chakra, Meridian, and Sports massage.

Senda pays special attention to your joints rather than to your muscles or to particular movements. The muscle strength will come as a by-product of tending to the joints. And to move the joints in all possible directions is the only way to make sure they get enough nutrients to stay functional. Keeping the joints flexible will keep the muscles and fascia flexible and balanced. When you start neglecting a joint, the muscles and fascia around it will be affected: one side will get contracted and the other one overstretched. This, in turn, will start affecting the next joint in the body. In case you keep ignoring the problem, it will extend to the farther parts of the body.

For example, the neglected left ankle will affect the left knee; the unbalanced left foot muscles and fascia will affect the left calf and thigh fascia and muscles. If you keep ignoring the left ankle, it will start affecting the left hip, the muscles and fascia in the left foot will affect the fascia and muscles up to the left lower back. In the end, all this will result in a contracted left side and over stretched right side of the body.

In the end, this book will teach you how to be aware of your body right here and right now, to balance your movements, and to improve your beautiful mechanism.

Why do you need to have this book?

The answer is simple, there are 2 reasons:

1. Because the body has joints.

2. Because you need to move from one place to another in this life, and because you need the movement to think, breath, drink, eat, etc.

What Senda will give you

You will gain insights into the general concept of Senda and examples of exercises for re-learning familiar movements and learning the new ones.

The exercises will help you understand your movements better, do them properly, and – most importantly – avoid injury and health problems that could result from unbalanced movements. That is what the many exercises are for. Still, these are examples. The more you understand the concept of Senda and apply it to all kinds of situations in your life, the more you will be able to create your own exercises and share your knowledge with others.

In other words, Senda:

- Brings you awareness of your movements

- Simplifies the complex

- Shows you in detail how the movement happens

- Complements other sport activities – how to get in and out of the exercise

- Relieves the pain caused by neglecting and slowly injuring and overusing parts of your body

- Minimizes the risk of injury at any time, especially when you do not expect it

- Guides you on your path to creating a mindset of motion, balance, and improvement.

- How important the Gatekeepers (jaws, neck, shoulders and hips) are, and how they talk to you when they have a problem or when one of your organs has a problem.

- To use Zero Technique to help the channels of the Gatekeepers to stay clean.

- Senda will make you think differently about everything.

Once your mind is familiar with Senda, you do not need to limit yourself to these exercises. To the contrary: my goal is that you create your own exercises using Senda Principles to keep your body in balance.

Read this book section by section. Get comfortable with one section before moving on to the next one.

p.s. If you have pain, injury, or illness, even if it is in one of your internal organs, do the second part of the book (starting from Basics of lifestyle) first and the first part of the book second.

Senda's insights

Senda tells you to never settle and never do the same thing every day again. Routine is good on a high level – such as running every day. But on a detailed level, running routine is toxic because you only run forward using the same muscles and moves. According to Senda, you should walk forwards, sidewards and backwards using your steps in different creative ways.

Senda wants you to embrace many ways of moving, many poses and all muscles. So be aware of your **joints** and switch the poses, the moves, the way of doing things. Always do something but always change the way you do it. Stop asking yourself whether the movement you are making is right and healthy. Everything is right and correct but do not hold on to a particular movement, keep on changing. Move **intentionally** all the time (stretch, shift your weight, move just a single part of your body) – until you start doing it subconsciously.

Learning Senda is like learning how to drive a car: In the beginning, you may be overwhelmed by all the information and detail, but ultimately you do it automatically. This becomes especially important when you are focusing on something, for example studying or working on a project. At this time, you are not paying attention to what your body is doing.

Example 1: When you are sitting at the desk, your shoulder(s) go up and your back gets curved automatically. These are not natural positions for the joints. You have to bring your shoulders to the exact opposite, hold for a while, then start moving your shoulders in different ways.

Example 2: If you have an office job and you use the right hand for the mouse, check your wrist. You will see that your hand is in Flex position (see page 95). After learning what the Zero position for the wrist is, you need to bring your right hand to the exact opposite of your previous position. Then, start moving your hand in all possible directions while you are still using it in your work.

Example 3: If you have your shoulders leaned forward while studying, standing or working, learn what the Zero position of the shoulders is and bring them to the exact opposite of your previous position. Keep doing your activities, then start moving the shoulders in all possible directions.

Example 4: Running can be dangerous if it is done unbalanced. In fact, the harm from keeping your ankles unbalanced while running may outweigh the advantages of this nice activity. You have to keep your ankles in the middle unless you are rolling the ankles in/out consciously on purpose.

By doing this, you will improve the quality of your own life and also have a chance of improving the life of others.

to move

it's too late

before

Move

Move in balance before imbalance moves you in pain

You might ask yourself:

Why should I do Senda? Is Senda something for me? Do I need to do Senda?

Yes!

Make your own choices; use your free will to move your body with Senda – otherwise the circumstances will force you to move it later (when your body gets problems from being neglected).[1] In other words, preventing health problems is always better than treating them!

---

[1] Consider the following example. Imagine you do not pay enough attention to your shoulders and neck as you never stretch them and do not build the necessary muscles supporting them. Your shoulders and neck are then not prepared for many different movements you might expose them to without even being aware of that. It is highly likely that some of these movements will give you pain – you will need to visit a doctor then. But a doctor will treat you with physiotherapy and massage – so you will be forced to move under her prescription rather than on your own will.

Remember: Everyone came and comes to this life at the exact time when something special is to be delivered.

Don't wait for the right time to give others the missing part of what they need, make NOW the right moment.

Contents

Essential Senda techniques

No matter in which position you are (sitting, standing, walking, training, etc.), use the following techniques without changing your position.

Sandwich

Engage both your lower/middle abdominals and lower/middle back muscles and push your stomach (especially your lower stomach) to your lower back without moving the shoulders or hips. Find this position by laughing or coughing. It should feel like you are squeezed a bit like a sandwich from front and back. Apply this technique when you are sitting, walking, running, driving, cleaning, etc. throughout your day. How exactly you apply this technique may vary: hold it for a few seconds or for a few minutes; repeat in a set of 3 times or 11 times.

Spreading

Spread your fingers, then circle your wrists. Do this before, during and after an activity in which you use your hand(s), for example, in writing, cleaning, lifting, doing sports.

Spread your toes, then circle your ankles. Do this before, during and after an activity in which you use your feet, for example, in sitting, standing, walking, biking, driving, doing sports.

This technique will balance the parts of your body used in these activities.

Breathing

Take 2 minutes to breathe consciously. Use your own technique to make a deep inhale and a deep exhale.

I recommend inhaling deeply through the nose while also using the muscles around your ribs and stomach. Hold your breath for a few seconds, then exhale deeply and as slowly as you can from your mouth using your rib and stomach muscles again. As an option, hold your breath for a few seconds also after exhaling. Use your hand to close your nose pretending that you are trying to inhale while you are holding your breath. Then, exhale further through your mouth. Repeat this at least three times before inhaling again.

Challenge yourself every day by holding your breath for 1 minute at least. This is a daily reboot for your body that refreshes you and increases your endurance.

When you hold your breath, you give your lungs more time to absorb oxygen-rich (O_2) air and release carbon dioxide-rich (CO_2) air. It stimulates your blood circulation and in the long term increases your lung capacity, protects your brain cells.

Zero Position

According to Senda principles, the Zero Position is a natural body pose rather than an exercise. It is natural because you only need minimum energy to keep it. You achieve it by aligning your body parts with each other optimally.

Big toes, feet and knees

While standing, walking or running, the body weight is carried by the feet. You should always keep your big toe, foot, ankle, and knee aligned. After bringing the big toe to the center (defined as a position in which your big toe looks in the same direction as your foot), check if the ankle is rolled-in (eversion) or rolled-out (inversion). You need to bring it to the middle.

Once you have your big toe and ankle fixed (centered), the feet and knees will align automatically. That is, you will have your knees parallel when your feet are parallel, and your knees turned out/in when your feet are turned out/in.

To bring your legs to Zero Position, you need to put your feet at hip-width. To find your hip-width,

First, bring your feet together.
Second, turn out your right foot so that it is at 90 degrees to your left foot.
Third, make Point with your right foot and raise your heel up without moving the tip of your right big toe.
Fourth, turn your right foot to make it parallel to the left one while keeping the right foot in Point.
Fifth, put your right foot down keeping it parallel to the left one without moving the tip of your right big toe.
Sixth, slide your right foot to the front (keep it parallel to the left one) till it is on the same level with the left foot.

> **Flex**: A flexed foot is one where the heel is actively pushing away from the body while the top of the foot with the toes pull upwards and towards the body.
> **Point**: Pointing is the opposite action of flexing, as the toes now actively push away from the body.

Zero Position for feet, ankles and knees should be used while walking, climbing stairs, walking down stairs, running, and doing any sports that involve bending knees. The reason is that there is a lot of pressure on the knees and ankles during such activities.

If the big toe, the ankle and the knee are not aligned, either foot or knee will eventually get injured. Due to such a misalignment, you will also develop problems with your hips, back, or neck at some point.

Once you have your big toe and ankle fixed (centered), the feet and knees will align automatically.

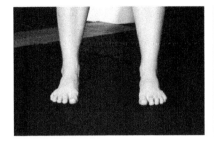 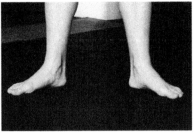 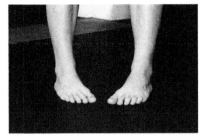

To bring your legs to Zero Position, you need to put your feet at hip-width. To find your hip-width,

First, bring your feet together.

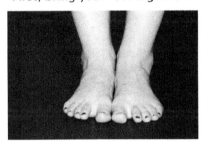

Second, turn out your right foot so that it is at 90 degrees to your left foot.

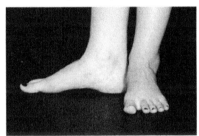

Third, make Point with your right foot and raise your heel up without moving the tip of your right big toe.

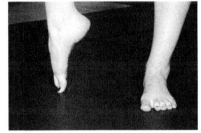

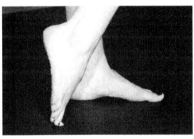

Fourth, turn your right foot to make it parallel to the left one while keeping the right foot in Point.

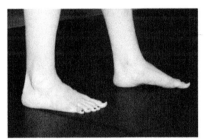

Fifth, put your right foot down keeping it parallel to the left one without moving the tip of your right big toe.

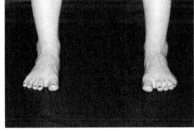

Sixth, slide your right foot to the front (keep it parallel to the left one) till it is on the same level with the left foot.

Flex: **Point**:

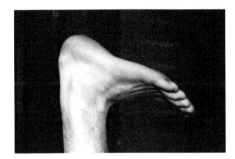 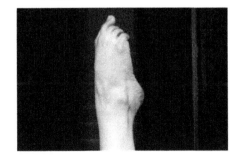

Hips

Control your hips! The Zero Position for the hips is their neutral position – in the middle. The following movements will help you to get to your middle. Move your hips to your maximum forwards (Cat) and backwards (Horse), then move your hips left and right. The middle (in both directions) is your neutral position.

Cat: A pose with your lower back rounded (flexion) and your hip joints brought forward.
Horse: A pose with your lower back arched (extension) and your hip joints brought backwards.

Ribs

The Zero Position for the ribs is having your ribs slightly pushed down. Find this position by laughing or coughing. Alternatively, imagine someone is suddenly hitting you in your stomach – you will push your ribs down in a natural reaction to such a hit (like a cat).

Wrists

To get to the Zero Position for your wrists, do the following. Put your hand and elbow on a table. Make a fist (without using your thumb), put the upper knuckles on the table. Your wrist will be slightly above the table. Your index finger will be able to fit tightly between your wrist and the table.

Elbows

To reach Zero Position for the elbows, you need to turn them in and out until you find the middle where the muscles are relaxed (not used).

Note: If you are writing or typing, you need to put your elbows on a base (not let them free in the air) and lean forward with your upper body. This way, your shoulders do not have to bear the weight of your arms. Therefore, you will not get problems with your wrists, arms, shoulders, or neck. Also, you do not have weight on your lower back and hence will not have problems with it either. But do not forget to keep changing to other positions!

Cat   **Horse**

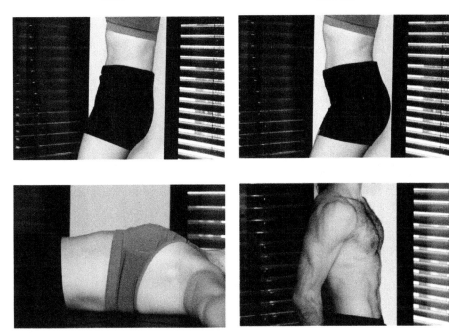

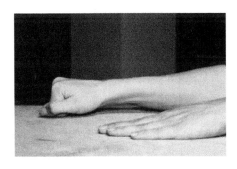

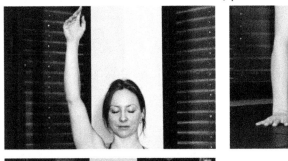

To get to the Zero Position for your wrists, do the following. Put your hand and elbow on a table. Make a fist (without using your thumb), put the upper knuckles on the table.

To reach Zero Position for the elbows, you need to turn them in and out until you find the middle

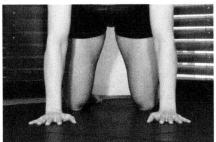

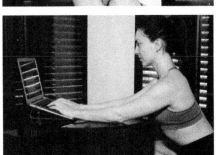

Note: If you are writing or typing, you need to put your elbows on a base (not let them free in the air) and lean forward with your upper body. This way, your shoulders do not have to bear the weight of your arms. Therefore, you will not get problems with your wrists, arms, shoulders, or neck. Also, you do not have weight on your lower back and hence will not have problems with it either. But do not forget to keep changing to other positions!

Shoulders

To determine your Zero Position, rotate your shoulders from up to back and down (backwards) and engage your latissimus, rib muscles and abs.

For example,

If your weight rests on your hands or elbows – like in All Fours, plank position, low plank position, handstand and similar exercises, the Zero Position for the arms is as wide as the shoulders.

To reach your shoulder-width, you can do the following:

1. Put your palms on the floor so that your wrists (their inner surface) are exactly below your shoulders (front surface).

2. Grab your left wrist with your right hand and put your right elbow on the floor so that your forearms form a 90-degrees angle.

3. Note where the outermost bit of your right elbow is.

4. Put your right palm on the floor in such a position that your thumb and index finger would embrace the right elbow if you kept it there.

5. Make sure your middle fingers point to the front. Open your fingers as far from each other as possible.

6. Push the tips of your fingers and the center of the palm against the floor.

7. Tune (turn) your elbows as indicated in the previous subsection.

Neck

Take a sitting or standing position, look to the front straight ahead. That might already be enough for you to make sure you have reached the Zero Position with your neck. If you are not sure, move your head to your maximum forwards and backwards (like a chicken) to find the middle. Make sure not to engage your jaw when you move your head forwards.

Jaws

The lower jaw must be in the middle. To find your middle, move your lower jaw to the right, to the left, back and front, every time reaching your maximum. It may help you to first bring the upper and lower front teeth (incisors) exactly over each other, and then move the lower jaw slightly backwards, letting it hang a bit.

To reach your shoulder-width, you can do the following:

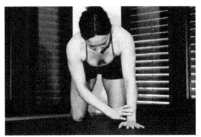

1. Put your palms on the floor so that your wrists (their inner surface) are exactly below your shoulders (front surface).

2. Grab your left wrist with your right hand and put your right elbow on the floor so that your forearms form a 90-degrees angle.

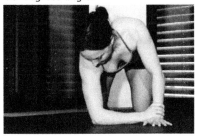

3. Note where the outermost bit of your right elbow is.

4. Put your right palm on the floor in such a position that your thumb and index finger would embrace the right elbow if you kept it there.

5. Make sure your middle fingers point to the front. Open your fingers as far from each other as possible.

6. Push the tips of your fingers and the center of the palm against the floor.

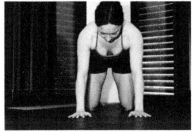

7. Tune (turn) your elbows as indicated in the previous subsection.

move your head to your maximum forwards and backwards (like a chicken) to find the middle

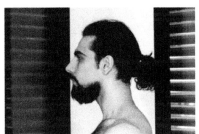

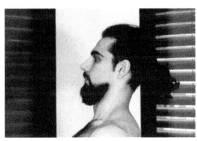

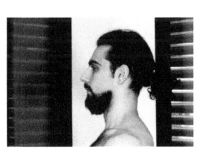

back and front, every time reaching your maximum

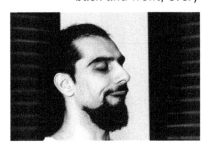

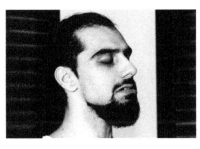

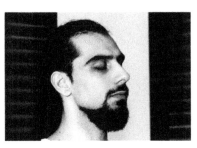

Summary

When a part of your body is going out of balance, you should bring it back to the Zero Position. Consequently, you need to pay attention to where your center of mass is, what body parts carry your weight.

The Zero positions can be applied in any situation, e.g., when lying, sitting, standing, walking, running, or doing sports.

Do not remain in one specific position for a long time. The elements of the Zero Position are important, indeed, but changing this position is as important.

Examples:

1. If you are sitting in a "comfortable" position (a position that you are probably used to and that does not follow Zero Position of Senda principles), for example, with a rounded or twisted back, it is not a problem. You simply need to keep on switching positions in order to keep your body flexible and functional for the longest period possible.

2. To keep the hips fit and healthy, switch between left, Cat, right, Horse and neutral positions in your own rhythm.

3. When lying down, minimize the tension in your lower back, make sure the hips are in their neutral position with the ribs slightly pushed down.

Move, and move before you move, and
move after you move

Daily routines

Throughout your day till this moment (till you read this book), you do many repeating moves without ever thinking about them. But you should start thinking about your moves.

Apply the following Guiding principles to every activity every day.

1. What am I doing right now?
2. Where is the weight resting? [2]
3. What is the exact opposite of the movement I am making?
4. How do I improve?

In the following, we provide examples of daily routines that can be optimized with some effort and thinking from your side. Practice them consciously until your body starts doing its own Senda without your mind controlling it. At this point, your routines have become Senda routines.

---

[2] By rest point of the weight we mean the center of mass.

Waking up

When you wake up, you need to gradually come back to this world from the place of dreams and recovery. It would not be wise to jump out of bed even if you felt fit enough. The body needs to adjust first, and your joints need a little warm-up before going to the active mode. Start to stretch your body like a tiger/cat when they wake up. Stretching like a tiger/cat is the way to tell your body that the new day has just started and it needs to be awake.

If you do not stretch the parts of your body which you are going to use during your day, the body will not be well-prepared to the challenges of the day.

Then, do a little warm-up that consists of small movements, starting with toes, ankles, slowly going to knees, hips, back, shoulders, elbows, wrists, fingers, mouth, eyes, and, finally, neck. Pay special attention to moving the joints in your feet, hands and jaws.[3] For example, for ankles, raise your legs and switch between Flex and Point with your feet, then turn them in circles as explained in subsection "Re-charging".[4] After this little warm-up, hug yourself (do a baby pose) – and you are ready to get up!

Be fair to your body, and you will not get illness or pain.

Standing up

If you *always* stand up the same way, it will lead you to an injury. This is because you are using the same set of joints and muscles in the same way every time, which makes your body unbalanced. The way you stand up is not incorrect; it is only unfair that you do it in the same way every time. You need to keep changing the way you stand up every day.

Examples:

1. Bring both legs to your chest first and then push them both towards the standing position.

2. If you are lying on your back, you have three options to change your position before standing up: (1) turn to your left side, (2) turn to your right side, or (3) turn around to your stomach. Choose a body part you want to stand on first: This could be hands, elbows, knees. For example, go into a handstand to get out of your bed.

---

[3] If you do such a warm-up regularly enough, the movements facilitating the activation of joints will become subconscious, automatic, and you might even be able to start doing Senda in your sleep.

[4] It is best to continue rotating until you get the feeling that your ankles got more flexible.

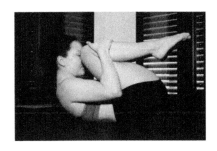 (do a baby pose)

and your joints need a little warm-up before going to the active mode. Start to stretch your body like a tiger/cat when they wake up

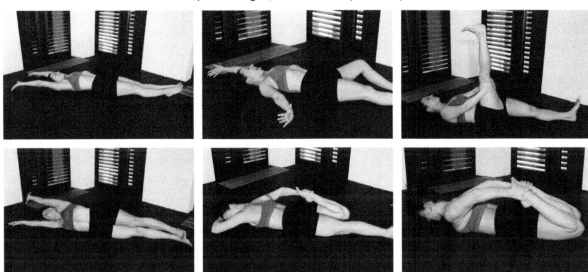

1. Bring both legs to your chest first and then push them both towards the standing position

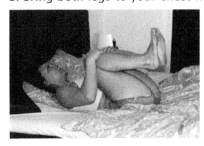 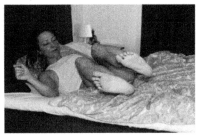 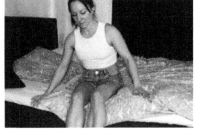

All Fours: Put the palms on the floor directed straight to the front, spread your fingers keeping the middle finger in the center. Press each knuckle down, especially those of index fingers. Your knees are under your hips and there is a 90 degrees angle between your back and thighs. Turn the inner elbows forwards without too much effort, the inner surface of your wrists is exactly below your shoulder (under the armpit) – follow the description of shoulder-width in Zero Position for Shoulders. In this position, your feet, knees and palms are on the floor, feet slightly flexed. Your neck is in line with your spine. Move your head while your eyes look to your knees till you can see the knees and a bit of your thigh. Then, look to the ground without moving your head. Now, push your neck and upper body up to the sky. Move your hips into a slight Cat till you feel the tension in your lower stomach and lower back.

A neutral way to stand up from the floor is to get to All Fours position first; then push your weight from your hands to your feet and roll up using Cat in your hips, lower back and middle back.

Use the reverse procedure to go down. For example, for picking something up from the floor, or for moving to the sitting/lying position. Make sure to land very softly with your hands and knees and keep in mind the Zero Position.

This way, you minimize the probability to get pain and functionality problems in ankles, knees, hips, lower back, neck and hands as time passes.

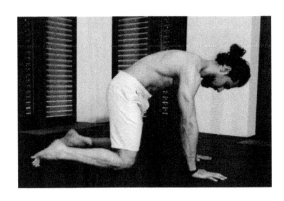 **All Fours**

A neutral way to stand up from the floor is to get to All Fours position first; then push your weight from your hands to your feet and roll up using Cat in your hips, lower back and middle back.

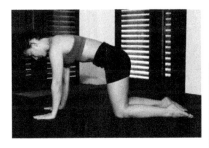

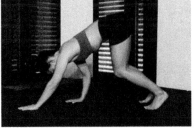

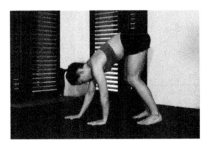

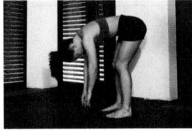

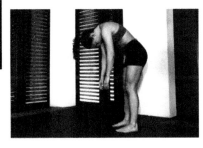

48

Don't leave your life –

           Live your life!

This routine takes from 1 to 11 minutes until you feel charged. We recommend you to take your time and enjoy it. When you have pain in some part of your body, just hold it there for a while till your joints and muscles come to their limits.[5]

1. Start with Zero Position in standing, feet at hip-width and parallel, hips in the middle, ribs gently pushed down and inwards, abs gently pushed down and towards your lower and middle back (think of the "Sandwich technique" when you do that).

2. Twist your neck: Bring it to Zero Position, then look to the right and slowly turn your head till you reach your maximum rotation. Hold few seconds. Then look to the left, slowly turn your head till you reach your maximum. Hold few seconds. Repeat this twist at least 6 times.

3. Circle your head. With a long neck, lean your head forward and down (push your chin down and towards your chest). First, move the head to the left (move the left ear to the left shoulder), hold the position for a few seconds. Then move your head backwards and hold this position for a few seconds. Next, move your head to the right (bring the right ear to the right shoulder) and hold for a few seconds. Then, move your head down and hold again. Make another circle in the same direction (so that you have made 2 circles in total). Change the direction and make 2 circles with your head again. At the end of this circle, you will find your face looking straight down, chin tucked in towards your chest.
Do the same again with your mouth opened to the maximum – you can use your wrist as a help to reach your maximum. Put your wrist between your teeth and start moving your head as explained before. This will release your jaws and muscles around them and in the neck until the shoulders. Among other benefits, it will help you to get rid of teeth gnashing.

Flow: Smooth, steady and continuous motions like the steady flow of a river.

4. Keep your head down. Bring your shoulders forwards as far as you can and raise them to the ears; hold a few seconds. Then bring your shoulders to the middle keeping them raised and hold a few seconds. Then bring your shoulders backwards while still keeping them raised. Hold a few seconds. Finally, lower your shoulders while keeping them backwards. Start raising your head and circle your shoulders at least two times in a Flow: Start forward, then up, then backwards, and, finally, down.

---

[5] This will make your body ready to move freely.

Do the same again with your mouth opened to the maximum – you can use your wrist as a help to reach your maximum

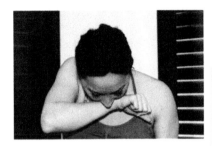
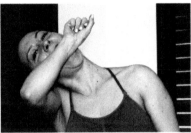
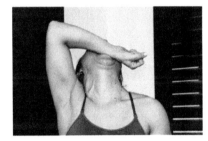
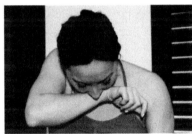
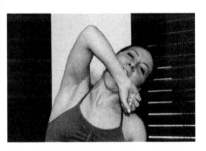

5. Bring your elbows as close as possible to the sides of your body and keep them there. Make your hands parallel to each other and clench your fists. The thumb should be on the side, not up and not inside your fist. Start circling outwards with your forearms without rotating them. Slowly do at least two circles. Make sure your wrists are in Zero Position.

Lony and Rony: Lony is the left little finger and Rony is the right little finger.

6. Make circles with your whole arms outwards. Start with your arms shoulder-wide and keep this distance while bringing your arms as far up and backwards as possible. As you reach the highest point with your hands, turn your shoulders, arms and palms out (start the rotation from Rony and Lony) to your limit. As you bring your arms down behind your back (shoulder-wide), turn everything in, shoulders, arms, palms (start again from Rony and Lony), and repeat the whole circle again. Do the circling at least two times in a slow Flow.

   This exercise is very important because a lot of your daily movements are the opposite of this routine – you hold your shoulders raised and forward, for example, if you are carrying a backpack or sitting and writing.

7. Keep your upper body and legs straight. Bring your hips to Zero Position. Twist your upper body, first turning slowly to the right till you reach your maximum. Hold few seconds. Then twist slowly to the left till you reach your maximum. Hold few seconds. Repeat this twist, but make it wider engaging your hips and legs. Keep your ankles in the middle.

8. Start with your back straight and bend your knees (Demi-plié). Make sure your hips are over the heels. Keep your knees bent; move the hips to Horse and then to Cat. Next, go wider, move with your chest and back switching between Horse and Cat. This is a very useful exercise – especially if you sit a lot, e.g., driving a car, but also if you walk a lot or use a repeating movement at work.

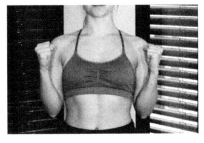 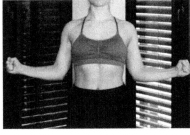

5. Bring your elbows

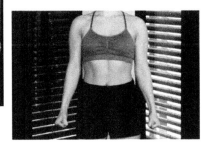

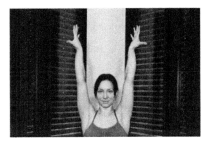 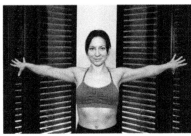

6. Make circles

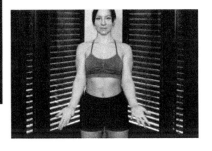

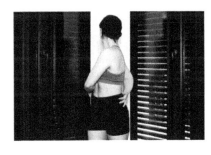 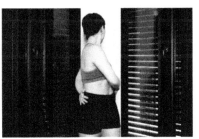

7. Keep your upper

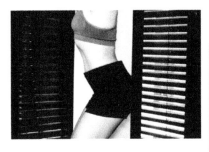 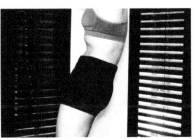

8. Start with your

> **Demi-plié**: A ballet pose in which you bend the knees halfway, keeping the heels securely on the ground. Your ankles are in the middle (neither rolled in nor rolled out).

> **Wave**: A body movement that reminds a wave on a water surface.

9. Do a Wave starting with your head facing downwards. Follow with your neck, shoulders, chest, and lower back, and hips in Cat. Next, do Horse with your hips and make your upper body horizontal like a table.

   Pay attention that

   a) your neck is in line with your back as explained in All Fours box;

   b) your head is pushing forwards and your hips are pushing backwards;

   c) your hips are over the heels.

   Hold the position for a few seconds, then drop down towards the floor. Let your upper body fall forward and feel heavy.

10. Roll up in the reverse Wave: Move your hips, making Cat, then the Wave continues in the lower back and the chest. Feel every vertebra in your spine. Continue the Wave rolling back up with your shoulders, neck and, finally, head. Hold your head back for a few seconds and turn your Lony and Rony in (arms out), shoulders following, until you feel tension in your shoulders. Hold a few seconds.

11. Roll down as in the first part of 9. without making a table with your upper body.

12. Do the plank. To do it, you need to follow the following steps.

    First, do All Fours. Tense every muscle and, focused, slowly start pushing from your heels backwards till your legs are straight. Do a slight Cat with your Hips in order to have a straight line from head to heels.

    Challenge yourself to bring your whole body as far to the front as you can.

Hold your plank for a few seconds. Breathe using your own technique or the technique described in "Essential Senda techniques"

Demi-plié

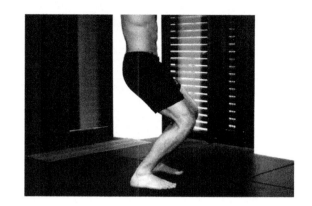

9. Do a Wave starting with your head facing downwards

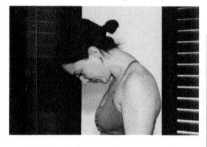
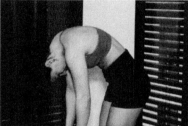
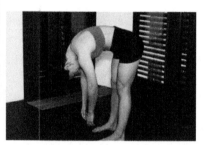
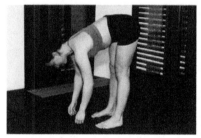
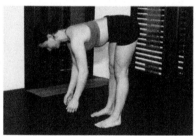
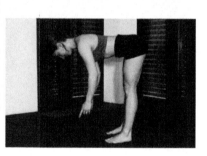

12. Do the plank. To do it, you need to follow the following steps

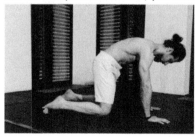
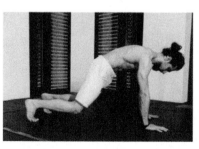
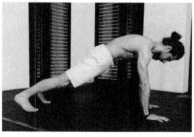

13. Put your knees down to the floor, exactly below your hips. Then bring your hips slightly backwards and do a slight Cat. Lay your forehead and nose softly on the floor; the backs of your hands are facing the floor with the fingers pointing to your feet. Bring the elbows as close to your body as you can. Hold for a while. If you do not feel much stretch in your wrists, bring the hands closer to your head, actively push your shoulders to the Zero Position. Hold it a few seconds till you feel that is enough.

14. Do high-five with the floor, then sit on your shins with your feet in Point. Bring knee to knee and hold your pointed feet at the same distance between them as between your knees. Keep your ankles in the middle and feet parallel (straight). If you have a knee problem, use one or more pillows between your calf and your thigh.

    Open your chest without doing Horse with your back. Use the "Sandwich technique" for your ribs. Then straighten your arms to both sides. Start rotating Rony and Lony in, elbows and shoulders following (keep your shoulders in zero position). Imagine you are drilling two holes with your arms in the two walls on your sides. Hold a few seconds. Move your head diagonally up.

15. Keep the same pose as in 14. and move your feet slowly from Point to Flex. Start rotating Rony and Lony outwards, elbows and shoulders following. Again, imagine the drilling picture above. Tuck your chin in. Hold a few seconds.

16. Finish the exercise by getting to All Fours, push your hips back and roll up as in 10. In the end, let your head softly fall back and rotate Lony and Rony in, arms and shoulders following. Hold the position in your limit for a few seconds.

Feel free to alternate this warm up with two modifications:

1- Follow the steps till and including 8. while standing on one leg or switching the legs from one to another. From step 9. on, do everything normally.

2- Do the steps till and including 11. with your back on the floor to find new positions of pain to work on. From step 12. on, do everything normally. At the end, do step 16. on your back.

NOTE: Every time you hold a pose for a few seconds, take a deep inhale and make a deep exhale using your own technique or the technique described in "Essential Senda techniques".

13. Put your knees down to the floor, exactly below your hips. Then bring your hips slightly backwards and do a slight Cat. Lay your forehead and nose softly on the floor;

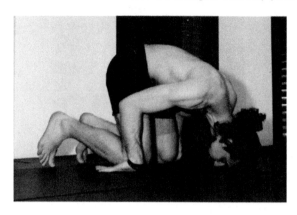

14. Do high-five with the floor, then sit on your shins with your feet in Point.

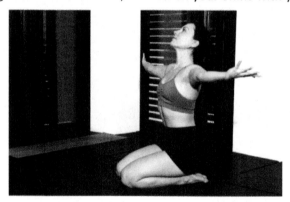

15. Keep the same pose as in 14. and move your feet slowly from Point to Flex.

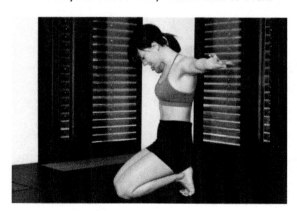

The ocean is dark, but not black.

Be like the ocean and the shelter

For everyone around you,

even if they say:

You are black inside.

What am I doing?

I am sitting. Examples include relaxed sitting on a sofa, sitting at your desk and writing/typing, putting your makeup on, having a meal, or going to the toilet.

Where is the weight resting?

The weight is on your hips and lower back. The weight could also be on the ankles, or on your elbows.

What is the exactly opposite movement?

Use the same distance and the same angle in the opposite direction

Check your ankles: are they rolled-in, rolled-out, or in the middle? If they are not in the middle, make the opposite of rolled-in or rolled-out.

If your hips and lower back are in Cat, bring them to Horse, and vice versa.

In case your shoulders are in a raised forward position, push them back and down.

If your chin has moved closer to your chest (down), raise it while keeping your gaze where it was.[6] After a few seconds, bring your neck backwards still keeping the gaze where it was.

For example: In case your weight is on the right side of your body (or your right arm, right elbow), bring your shoulder in the exactly opposite direction. You are probably holding your shoulders a bit forward and upward – push it backwards and down. Continue pushing with your ribs to your left side and push with your elbow against the desk or sofa (depending on where you are sitting) to get your chest higher up to the left. Do the opposite for your neck: for example, if your neck was leaning to the right and forward, bring it to the left and backwards, and vice versa.

Feel free to do the opposite movements presented above simultaneously or one by one.

How do I improve?

Move your neck, shoulders, arms and upper body as described in "Re-charging", steps from 2 to 7.

---

[6] The angle between your chin and horizontal plane parallel to the floor should remain the same (but up rather than down).

If your hips and lower back are in Cat, bring them to Horse, and vice versa.

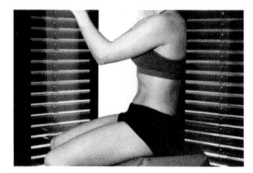 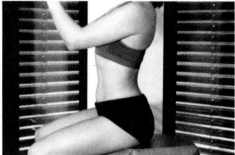

If your chin has moved closer to your chest (down), raise it while keeping your gaze where it was

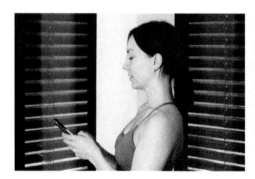 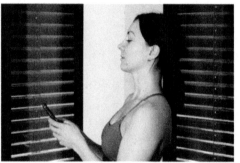

For example: In case your weight is on the right side of your body (or your right arm, right elbow), bring your shoulder in the exactly opposite direction. You are probably holding your shoulders a bit forward and upward – push it backwards and down. Continue pushing with your ribs to your left side and push with your elbow against the desk or sofa (depending on where you are sitting) to get your chest higher up to the left.

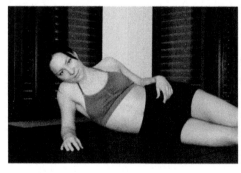 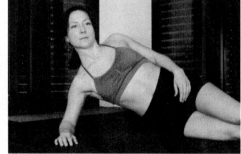

Sitting still for a prolonged period of time will make some parts of your body "fall asleep". This means your blood is not flowing enough in the parts that you are using for sitting, and the joints you use are constrained. To improve your blood circulation and your sitting pose, use the "Sandwich technique" described in Section "Essential Senda techniques" from time to time.

If you are working, reading, doing something with your phone, or sitting on the toilet, start moving your hips, alternating between Horse and Cat. Move your hips to the left and alternate between Cat and Horse again slowly. Move your hips to the right and repeat changing from Cat to Horse. In addition to the hips, move your feet (Relevé / Flex). Do this continuously – not fast at all. As an example, do Horse with your back – hold for a while – do Relevé with your feet and hold it. Do not rush and do not keep still.

> **Relevé**: The position of the foot with heels up and weight on the front part of the foot, more on the big toe than on the little toe.

Use a soft pillow behind your lower back and hips to prevent them from doing too much Cat. Feel free to keep the pillow behind while doing exercises described below.

Example 1. Circle your feet in the same direction slowly. Make a couple of circles, first starting left-upwards, then in the opposite direction.

Example 2. Move your hips in a circle while also shifting your weight. Start from left, then do Horse, then right, then Cat – then do it all over again a few times. Then do the circling in the opposite direction: Start from left, then do Cat, then right, then Horse. Do it slowly. Since your hips carry most of your weight when you are sitting, do this exercise as long as you are sitting.

Example 3. If you are sitting and writing for a prolonged time (for work or for studying), put your elbows on a support (do not let them "hang in the air" freely/unsupported) and lean with your upper body forward. Otherwise, you may get problems with your wrists, arms, shoulders, or neck. Challenge yourself by writing with the hand that you are not usually using for writing. Do the same with other activities you usually perform with your stronger hand, e.g., using the computer mouse.

Example 4. Do this as a quick break from sitting and a recharge for your back and legs. Bring your legs straight to the front while keeping the feet wider than hip-width. Feel free to switch between flexing and pointing your feet. Bring your upper body forward towards your legs until you reach your personal limit. Hold in that position for a while before rolling back up. Lean backwards and raise your arms behind your head. Feel free to straighten your arms.

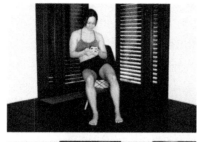 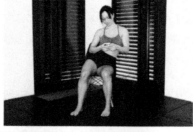

Move your hips to the left and alternate between Cat and Horse again slowly. Move your hips to the right and repeat changing from Cat to Horse

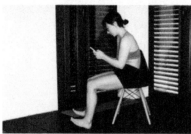 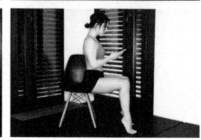

do Horse with your back – hold for a while – do Relevé

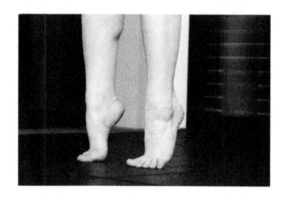

Relevé

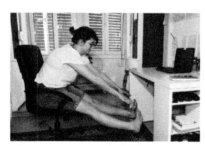 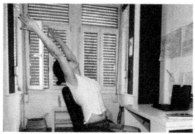

Example 4. Do this as a quick break from sitting and a recharge for your back and legs.

Example 5. Bring your leg to the side and keep it straight. Use an object to support your leg. Keep on with your activity (studying or working). Use different options, like straightening your leg to the front or to the back.

Example 6. Bring your legs to the sides and keep them straight. Use objects next to you to support your legs. Open your legs to 70% of your maximum. After a few moments, switch to a front split. Feel free to circle your hips while doing your 70%-splits. Start from left – Cat (see Example 2). Change the direction only once.

Example 7. While sitting, bring your feet to hip-width (see Hips) and raise your heels. Turn your feet in so that your knees touch each other. Stay in this position for a few moments. Turn your feet out while keeping the heels as high as they were and turn your knees out. Hold this position for a few seconds before putting the heels back down.

Example 8. While sitting, bring your feet and knees together. Without moving your upper body, bring your legs to the left in a twist – hold few seconds, then do the right side.

Example 9. If you are not writing or busy on your desk, put your right foot on your left thigh and gently move your right knee downwards. Reach for the ground with your hands over your leg. Put your whole palms on the ground if you feel bored.

Example 10. Pretend your pen has fallen down and stand up to pick it up. Next, move your hips a few times.

Example 11. Stand up and pretend you are curious about what is going on with your chair (is it mad or depressed because I was sitting on it for too long, or something else?). Lift the chair if you can, examine it, then put it slowly down. How to properly lift things is explained in the later section "Lifting, carrying and putting something down".

Example 12. If you cannot lift your seat (e.g., because it is heavy, fixed to the floor, a bench or a sofa), go to low push-up pose, hold there, check what is under your seat, then do a high push-up. Feel free to repeat this set of movements.

Example 13. Stand on your left leg and put your right foot on your seat if possible (take off your shoes if necessary), or on another object close to you. Feel free to move your hips between Cat and Horse, right and left; circle your hips few times. Start from left – Cat (see Example 2). Change the direction only once.

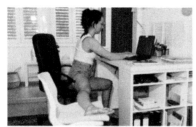 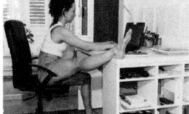 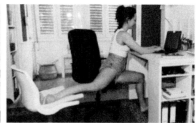

5. Bring your leg to the side and keep it straight. Use an object to support your leg. Keep on with your activity (studying or working).

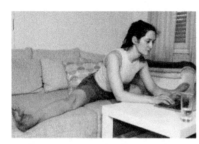 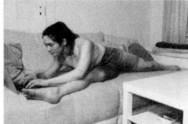 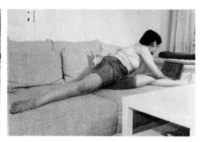

6. Bring your legs to the sides and keep them straight. Use objects next to you to support your legs. Open your legs to 70% of your maximum.

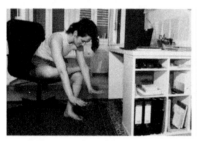 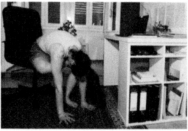

9. If you are not writing or busy on your desk, put your right foot on your left thigh and gently move your right knee downwards.

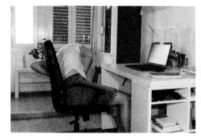 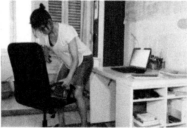 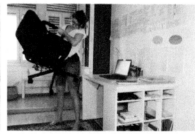

11. Stand up and pretend you are curious about what is going on with your chair (is it mad or depressed because I was sitting on it for too long, or something else?)

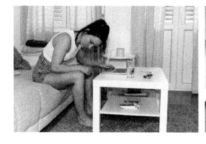 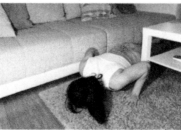

12. If you cannot lift your seat (e.g., because it is heavy, fixed to the floor, a bench or a sofa), go to low push-up pose, hold there, check what is under your seat, then do a high push-up.

Example 14. Bend your left leg and sit on your left shin[7] (use a pillow between your shin and your thigh if necessary) and do your best to reach the ground with your left knee. If your seat allows you to reach the floor, put your knee down or use a pillow in case you have pain without. The right leg is in front and 90 degrees bent in the knee (the angle between your foot and your shin is 90 degrees as well) – you will see that your knee is over your heel. Hold this position for a while, then take your seat again and straighten your left leg while raising it until it is parallel to the ground. Flex your foot while doing the last movement.

Example 15. When you are putting your make-up on, follow the techniques described in the examples above. Challenge yourself to use the hand you are not normally using while putting the make-up on.[8]

Example 16. While doing your hair, circle your shoulders backwards. Use any of the examples above while doing your hair whenever possible.

Example 17. When you are sitting because you are eating or drinking, use the examples above to introduce more dynamics to this pleasant activity. Switch between standing and sitting when you are having a drink. Constantly switch the hand you are using for grabbing the food. Before and after eating, move your neck, shoulders, arms, hips in all directions considering the joint movement and not your possible directions! Also move your upper body and legs. Do not be shy and try out Example 11 above.

Example 18. Challenge yourself to put your seat aside and do a squat ("sit in the air") on one or both legs. Follow the Zero Position principles for your big toes and ankles. Feel free to use a wall or another similar object as a support for your back. If you are squatting on one leg, feel free to put another leg – crossed – on your standing leg.

Example 19. Open your legs much more than hip-width and go into Second Position in dance with your feet turned out (make sure your big toe, foot, ankle and knee are aligned). Lean forward, put your bent arms on some surface at the level of your pelvis, the elbows are under the shoulders. Push your knees outside (backwards) and bring them back to where they were. Repeat the movement of the knees a few times. Once you reach the point where the pain becomes unbearable, hold the knees for few seconds.

> **Second Position in dance**: The feet can be turned in, turned out or parallel and spaced so far apart that the angle between shin and thigh is 90 degrees. It is allowed to bring your hips closer to the floor.

---

[7] Your left foot will likely find itself under your buttocks.
[8] Make sure there is enough light in the room not to strain your eyes.

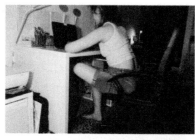 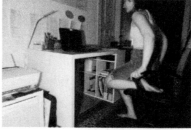 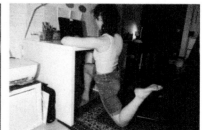

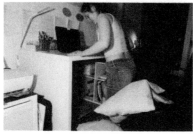 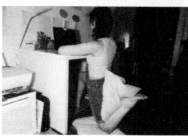

14. Bend your left leg and sit on your left shin (use a pillow between your shin and your thigh if necessary) and do your best to reach the ground with your left knee. If your seat allows you to reach the floor, put your knee down or use a pillow in case you have pain without.

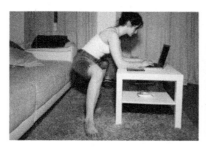 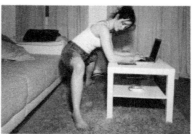

19. Open your legs much more than hip-width and go into Second Position in dance with your feet turned out (make sure your big toe, foot, ankle and knee are aligned). Lean forward, put your bent arms on some surface at the level of your pelvis, the elbows are under the shoulders.

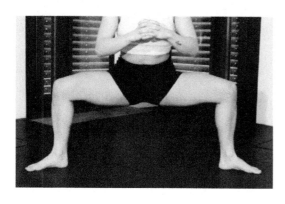

Second Position in dance

Example 20. If you are reading a book or using your smartphone or tablet while sitting, circle your hands reaching a maximum angle in your wrists. Follow the examples above and consider doing the following movements from time to time[9]:

    a. Rotate your shoulders and arms as described in "Re-charging".

    b. Move your face away from the screen (or from the page). Pretend someone is calling you from your right side – and follow the call with a rotation of your head. Circle your neck few times as described in "Re-charging". Bring your head backwards so that you look up and back – someone important is calling you from behind to see your beautiful face.

    c. Change the hand typing/holding the book or the smartphone.

    d. Lift your book or smartphone up in the air and slightly backwards – pretend you want to give it to someone sitting on the roof. Hold it a few seconds. Feel free to keep your arm straight or bent.

    e. Increase the distance between your book/smartphone and your eyes and keep reading. Allow a minute or two in this position before bringing your object back to its usual place. Bring your head up/down and keep your eyes on the same point where you were reading. Look at your screen or page from the side (use your eyes at all possible angles). These movements are activating the muscles around your eyes which became lazy because you did not use them.

Example 21. If you are sitting while putting on and off your socks and shoes, use the examples above whenever possible. Stretch your socks in all directions as much as you can. If the socks are tight and are squeezing your toes to each other, your joints will be pressed closer to each other than they should be – that will make the joints in your knees, hips, shoulders and neck stiff. After you have put on your socks and shoes, raise your legs one by one to your maximum keeping the knees straight.

Example 22. While sitting on the toilet, do not forget to follow the examples described above whenever possible. Start by circling the hips (Example 2). If time allows, continue with other examples.

---

[9] Actually, it would be good to do these movements (a break for your body from the working pose) as often as possible.

20.

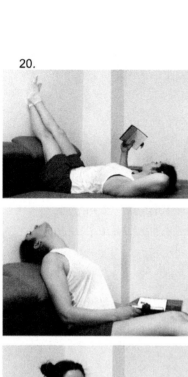 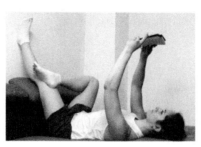 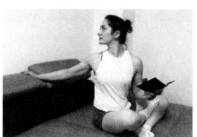

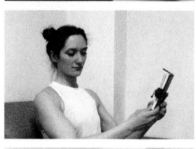

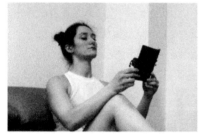 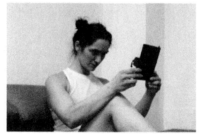

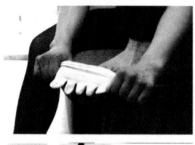 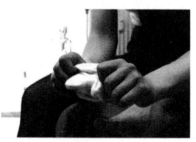

21.

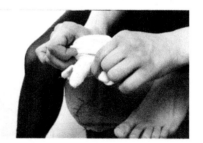

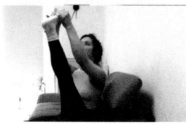 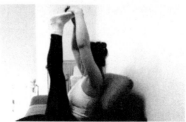

Change the way you stand up from sitting.

Example 1. Bring your feet to hip-width, keep your ankles in the middle. Keep your buttocks at your sitting level and slide forwards from your seat. Your knees go forwards and you end up in Demi-plié. Now, stand up.

Example 2. Start the movement as in Example 1. Instead of standing up immediately, make a few steps forwards gradually going up (taking off as an airplane). Shift your weight from one foot to another on each step. Take at least 3 steps before you get to your normal standing position. Feel free to choose the direction of your feet but keep your ankles in the middle.

Example 3. Cross your feet putting the left foot in front. Make a twist to the left with your upper body and stand up. Make sure to keep your ankles in the middle.

Example 4. Turn around while standing up. Now your face is in the opposite direction from where it was when sitting.

Example 5. Use All Fours to stand up from the floor as in subsection "Standing up"

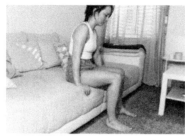 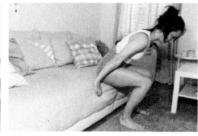 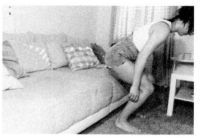

1. Bring your feet to hip-width, keep your ankles in the middle. Keep your buttocks at your sitting level and slide forwards from your seat.

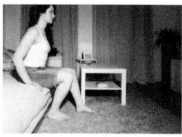 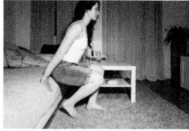 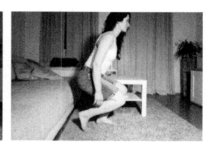

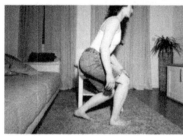 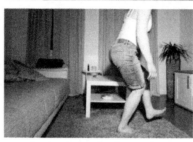

2. Start the movement as in Example 1. Instead of standing up immediately, make a few steps forwards gradually going up (taking off as an airplane). Shift your weight from one foot to another on each step.

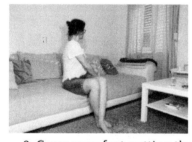 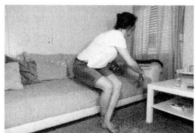 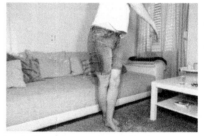

3. Cross your feet putting the left foot in front. Make a twist to the left with your upper body and stand up.

4. Turn around while standing up.

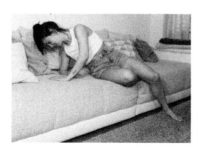 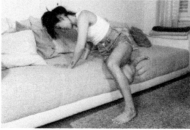 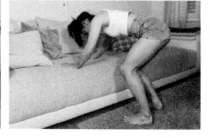

73

To Balance things, you need

To be unbalanced

What am I doing?

I am standing. Examples of situations in which you are standing include talking to someone, waiting for the traffic light, taking the elevator, standing in the public transport, washing your hands.

Where is the weight resting?

The weight is on your ankles and feet. The weight could also be on any other joints of your body that are used to support you, for example the back or shoulder if you are leaning on a wall with it.

What is the exact opposite of the movement I am making?

Use the same distance and the same angle in the opposite direction

Check your ankles whether they are rolled-in, rolled-out, or in the middle. If the ankles are not in the middle, do the exactly opposite of their current state – roll the ankles in or out. Bring your hips to the left if they were on the right side, into Cat if they were in Horse, and vice versa. If your shoulder is raised, lower it down to the same extent as it was up.

Apply the same principle on your neck, elbows and wrists, but only if you have weight on them. For example, if your neck is leaned forward and to the left, bring it first backward, hold it few seconds, then move it to the right. Note that the final position is symmetric to the starting position.

How do I improve?

Move your neck, shoulders, arms and upper body as described in "Re-charging", steps from 2 to 7.

You should always change the way you stand. Make sure to come back to Zero Position (Big toes, ankles, knees, hips, shoulders, neck) from time to time.

If you experience lower back pain from standing for a long time (also while you are cooking), bring your hips to Zero Position and engage both your lower/middle abdominals and lower/middle back muscles and push your stomach to your lower back without moving any other part of your body "Sandwich technique". Do this from time to time. Do this also to prevent pain in your lower back.

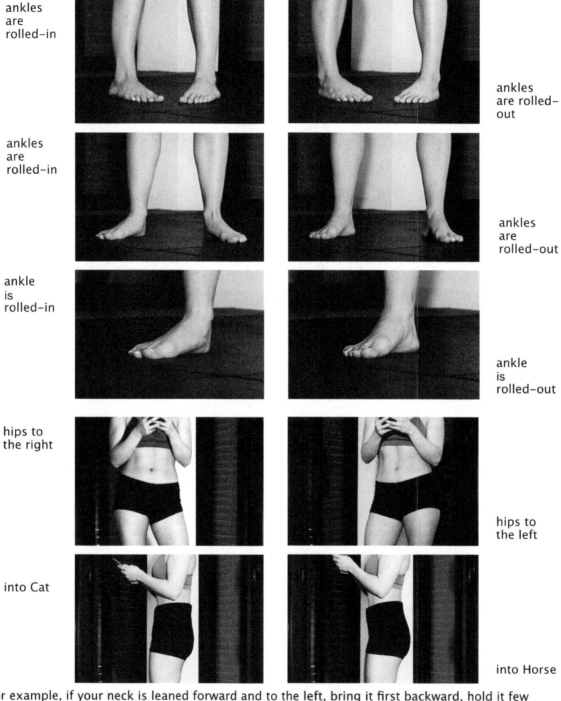

ankles
are
rolled-in

ankles
are rolled-
out

ankles
are
rolled-in

ankles
are
rolled-out

ankle
is
rolled-in

ankle
is
rolled-out

hips to
the right

hips to
the left

into Cat

into Horse

For example, if your neck is leaned forward and to the left, bring it first backward, hold it few seconds, then move it to the right. Note that the final position is symmetric to the starting position.

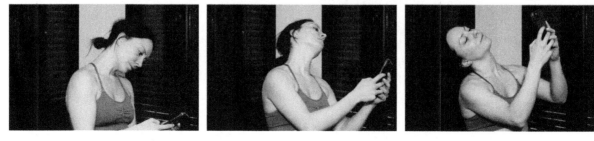

77

Example 1. From your own standing position, shift the weight from one foot to another. Switch between flexing and pointing your free foot (the one that does not support the weight) a few times. Rotate your free foot, first Anti-heartwise, and then Heartwise. Pay attention to keep the ankle of the standing leg in the middle.

Heartwise: the direction of circular movement from up (to the head) to the left, then down (to the feet), and then to the right.
Anti-heartwise: the direction of circular movement from up to the right, then down, and then to the left.

Example 2. Stand with your feet hip-width. Bend your knees while keeping them aligned with ankles and feet. You are free to keep your feet parallel, turned-in or turned-out. Hold a few seconds, then straighten your knees again. Repeat a few times. Once you are comfortable with that, start bending one knee only. You are free to suspend your leg in the air.

Example 3. Put your left foot to the side over a suitable object. Keep your right ankle in the middle and make sure you do not put weight on your left knee (be comfortable).

Start moving your hips in all directions (left, Horse, right, Cat). Then circle your hips Heartwise (left – Cat – right – Horse).

Example 4. Pretend something has fallen down – pick it up keeping your legs straight. Reach with your hands to the floor as much as you can. If you already can put your palms on the floor, do not stop there. Hold for a few seconds and then roll your upper body up as in step 10 of "Re-charging".

Example 5. Find an object to put your left foot on, in front of you. Choose a support for your foot in a height to your liking. Do not put too much weight on your left knee by leaning over it. Keep your heel on its place and start moving your left foot slowly and carefully to the left and to the right. Pay attention to your ankles – keep your ankles in the middle! You should feel some tension in your left thigh and in your left hip. Repeat a few times, then switch the leg.

Example 6. Bend your right leg while raising the right foot behind to your hip (buttocks). The right foot is Point and the ankle is in the middle. Keep the knees together and get hold of your right foot with one or both hands. Hold for a while. Release your hands and keep your bent leg at the same place, maybe enjoying a cramp in the muscle on the backside of your thigh. Hold for a few seconds, then bring the right foot down to the ground in front of you (at one step distance), Flex it and stretch by leaning forward with straight legs. Hold a few seconds. Do the whole exercise with your left leg as well.

Example 7. Raise one of your legs up to the side as high as you can. The other leg may be straight or bent, feel free to lift the heel of the standing leg up.

Example 8. Cross your feet keeping them together with the right one in front. Bend your upper body to the left side. Bring your right arm over your head and keep it straight. Put your left hand to the left hip and push it to the right. The left thumb is behind your back, the rest of the palm is directed forwards. You can do the same stretch keeping your feet apart. Increase the distance between your feet as you get more comfortable with this position.

Example 9. While standing in a shower, use the examples above whenever possible.

Example 10. Do you often use the same hand to open/close (push/pull) a door or to turn a key in a lock? If so, start using the other hand, do it for a while, and then start constantly switching the hand you are using. If you are carrying something and need to open/close the door, just drop the stuff beside you to the floor (using techniques explained below in subsection "Lifting, carrying and putting something down" Do not stress your body more than necessary!

Example 11. While putting your clothes on and taking them off, follow the examples described above and in the subsection "Sitting" Be creative in how exactly you put your clothes on or take them off – find different ways to do so. Before putting your clothes on or taking them off, do a small warm-up for the parts of your body that you are going to engage. For instance, if you are going to put a T-shirt on, circle your head, shoulders, arms, and also move your hips (check subsection "Re-charging" for details).

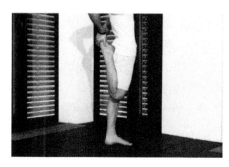

6. Bend your right leg while raising the right foot behind to your hip (buttocks). The right foot is Point and the ankle is in the middle. Keep the knees together and get hold of your right foot with one or both hands.

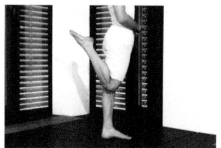

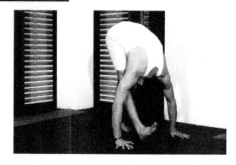

7. Raise one of your legs up to the side as high as you can. The other leg may be straight or bent, feel free to lift the heel of the standing leg up.

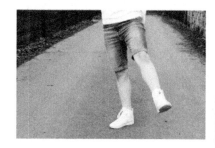

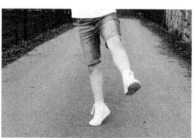

8. Cross your feet keeping them together with the right one in front. Bend your upper body to the left side. Bring your right arm over your head and keep it straight. Put your left hand to the left hip and push it to the right.

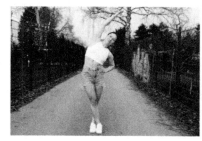

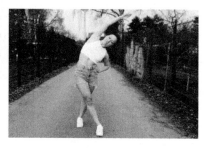

Example 12. While you are standing and cooking, do the exercises described above and "Sandwich technique". Also use the following suggestions:

1- Use the hand that you do not normally use for cooking.

2- While standing, turn your right foot out to the maximum. Hold a few seconds. Turn your right foot in to the maximum. Hold a few seconds. Make sure you keep your ankles in the middle. Repeat the same with your left foot.

3- Put small objects under your heels to bring them to a higher level than your toes (do not put on slippers or shoes). Hold for few minutes.

4- Sit for a while with one or both legs straight if possible.

Example 13. When you are putting your make-up on, follow the techniques described in the examples above. Challenge yourself to use the hand you are not normally using while putting the make-up on.[10]

Example 14. While doing your hair, circle your shoulders backwards. Use any of the examples above while doing your hair whenever possible.

There are many ways to keep moving while standing. The set of options available to you depends, of course, on your lifestyle, fitness, and the sports you are regularly practicing.

---

[10] Make sure there is enough light in the room not to strain your eyes.

The more you move,

the more you have to clean;

The less you move,

the more problems you get.

Whichever way you make your steps when walking, put your foot on the floor softly. Whether you start with your heels, sides or toes, roll softly to the rest of your foot.

To step softly, you have to use your leg muscles to bring your foot to the floor rather than stamp with it.

It is not incorrect to walk with your feet turned-in or out. It is, however, wrong, according to Senda, to repeat the same way of walking all the time.

All the three positions, parallel, turned-out, and turned-in, are correct, and need to be used recurrently when you are walking. It is, however, important in any of the 3 versions to keep your ankles in the middle. The exception is when you are rolling your ankles in or out on purpose to treat an injury or experience different ways of walking.

The things you need to be aware of while walking are the principles of Senda as described in Guiding principles

What am I doing?

I am walking.

Where is the weight resting?

There are two aspects to it.

The first aspect is what the ankles are doing. This is potentially the most important bit when it comes to walking. If the ankles are not in Zero Position, this costs energy and may create problems, as muscles are contracted to keep your ankle rolled-in or out.

The second aspect is the position of your upper body. This can be classified using the following four categories:

- Your upper body is leaning forwards, so it is leading your walking. Your hips do Horse or Cat. In any case, leaning forward makes your steps heavy and puts extra pressure on your hips and knees.

- Your upper body is leaning backwards; your hips automatically shift forwards. Your lower back muscles have to work a lot to keep this position.

- Your upper body is leaning to the side. This strains the muscles of your waist and puts additional pressure on the knee of the side to which you are leaning.

- Your upper body is in the middle, which is necessary for your Zero Position in walking.

What is the exact opposite of the movement I am making?

Use the same distance and the same angle in the opposite direction

Do the opposite of the movements that you do by walking. Since you are the one who knows best which walking style you are using, you know best the exact opposite of the movements you are doing.

The time you need to practice the opposite movement depends on how quickly your body adjusts to it. Once your body can do the opposite movement subconsciously, you are ready for the new ways to walk.

Example 1. If you are walking with your right foot turned-out and your ankle rolled-in, the opposite movement would be to turn your right foot in, keeping exactly the same angle between your right foot and the direction of your movement. Of course, you also need to roll the ankle out to the same extent.

Example 2. If you are walking with your hips doing Cat, you need to start walking with your hips doing Horse, and vice versa.

Example 3. If you are walking with your hips slightly twisted to the right (the left shoulder automatically leans forwards), you need to lean your shoulder backwards and twist your hips to the left.

Example 4. If your upper body is leaning forwards when you are walking, you need to start leaning backwards at the same angle relative to an imaginary vertical line, and vice versa. If your upper body is leaning to one side, start leaning to the other side.

Example 5. If you bend one of your knees and bounce it a lot when walking, start walking with an almost straight leg on the bouncing side. Later (after some weeks), start bouncing with the other leg while using the initial leg neutrally (without bending it too much, but also not straightening it completely). After some more weeks, start walking with straight leg on the side that was neutral initially.
Do not wonder that we recommend you to correct the side that was not bouncing. This is because the damage extends to the parts of your body other than legs and to neutralize it we need to work on the leg that was not initially affected.

If you are walking with your right foot turned-out and your ankle rolled-in,

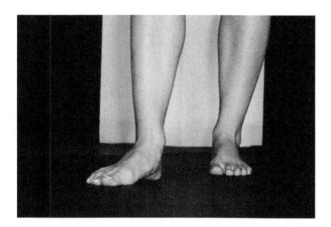

the opposite movement would be to turn your right foot in, keeping exactly the same angle between your right foot and the direction of your movement. Of course, you also need to roll the ankle out to the same extent.

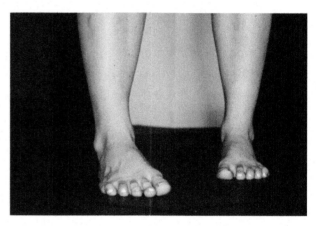

If you have pain (without any apparent cause) in your knees, hips, shoulders or neck when you are walking, doing the exact opposite as described above will lessen or eliminate your pain.

How do I improve?

Move your neck, shoulders, arms and upper body as described in "Re-charging", steps from 2 to 7.

Find new ways to walk. The examples below will give you an idea of how to do that. As a general rule, change the position of your hips between Horse, neutral, Cat, left, right.

If you experience lower back pain from walking for a long time, bring your hips to Zero Position and use the "Sandwich technique". Do this from time to time. Doing this will also prevent pain in your lower back.

Example 1. Look proud while walking: open your chest, bring your shoulders back and down.

Example 2. If you are dragging your foot with every step or often, this affects your ankles, knees, and hips. You need to lift your leg high enough with the move originating from your hip joint.

Example 3. Lift your left shoulder to your ear and walk normally. Then, twist to the right and walk further while still keeping your left shoulder raised. This walking style helps you to relieve pain on the left side of your lower back.
In case you have pain in your lower back (on both sides), raise both shoulders and walk. Switch between twisting your upper body left and right.

Example 4. Walk with tiny steps using your knees (lift your feet higher than usual). Make sure your ankles are in the middle however your feet are directed (parallel, turned-in or turned-out). Explore various options
- with your upper body (leaning forwards, backwards, to a side)
- with your neck (left, right)
- with the rhythm and speed (slow motion, fast, normal)

Example 5. Take steps that are larger than your usual steps. Explore the same options as in the example above. Make your steps grow larger and larger. Challenge yourself to reach your Lunge.

> **Lunge**: One leg is positioned forward with knee bent at 90 degrees or more and foot flat on the ground. The other leg is positioned behind with the foot as far backwards as possible. Ankles remain in the middle (not rolled-in or -out).

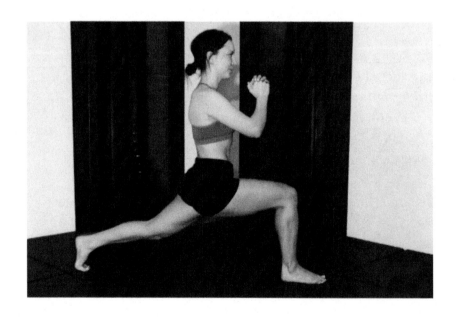

Lunge

Example 6. Lift your knees as high as you can while keeping your back straight. The movement should start from the hip and the hip is pulling your leg in. Do the same while twisting your upper body.

Example 7. Walk sideward crisscrossing your legs. Play with the distance: Take smaller and larger steps, change your leading leg. Change direction, experiment!

Example 8. Take small quick steps on the toes (in Relevé).

Example 9. You can stretch while walking when you step and straighten your knee to the maximum, and then push your thigh muscles backwards before making the next step. Do it slowly.

Example 10. Walk backwards using the same techniques as in the examples above. Note that you should start practicing walking backwards with your toes first. Later, you are free to use different methods.

Example 11. When you are cleaning, use your weaker hand for a couple of days or months until it becomes as strong as the stronger hand. Then, start alternating your hands and use them equally. While you are cleaning, follow the examples above and those from subsection "Sitting" to the extent possible, then also do the following moves:

1. Get to All Fours; if you are not comfortable with putting your knees on the floor, put something soft under them (a towel, a pillow).

2. Make some room between your feet by taking a long step in a direction of your choice. For example, you can make Lunge with your left leg. Continue cleaning.

3. Do the plank as described in "Re-charging". Continue cleaning with one hand. If it is too hard, put one of your knees down.

4. Take the Second Position, feel free to lean forward with your upper body and continue cleaning. Make sure to keep your ankles in the middle and feel free to choose the direction of your feet.

5. Use your feet instead of your hands to clean with.

Example 12. After-walking stretch: Use Example 6 in subsection "Standing"

The examples above give you an idea of how to create your movements and walking style. Before your muscles get fed up with walking the way you do, you have to stretch. You can walk and stretch at the same time, as the examples above show. After stretching as in Example 12, walk differently again.

Note: In case you carry something relatively heavy, please check the "Lifting, carrying and putting something down" and Wearing a backpack for more details.

Not every right movement

is correct and

not every wrong movement

is incorrect

What am I doing?

Using one side of my body (one hand, elbow, shoulder), I am lifting something, carrying it, and putting it down. The carrying part may involve walking on a plain ground, walking up or down stairs.

Where is the weight resting?

The weight is resting on the part of the body that is doing the lifting or carrying. If the thing you are carrying is touching your hips or your leg, the weight is also resting there.

What is the exact opposite of the movement I am making?

Use the same distance and the same angle in the opposite direction

If you do the lifting with your hand turned-in, start doing it with your hand turned-out, and vice versa. If you do the lifting or carrying with your elbow bent, you need to start doing it with your elbow straight. If you do the lifting with your shoulder up, bring your shoulder down; bring the shoulder backwards if it was forward.

So far, we have only paid attention to the parts of your body that you have directly used by lifting or carrying. Your toes, ankles, knees, hips, back, neck, and the free arm and shoulder however, may be used indirectly. Therefore, you need to do the opposite movement for each of the body parts that are engaged (put weight upon).

How do I improve?

Follow two principles to minimize the energy your muscles spend on lifting. First, keep your joints in Zero Position. Second, get as close as possible to the things you want to lift. The parts that are not actively carrying any weight should be brought to Zero Position. This is because Zero Position gives the optimal support for the active parts.

Use the weak side of your body to lift. Use different ways to lift things.

Before carrying something, circle your shoulders backwards, move your hands in every possible direction considering the joint movement and not your possible directions! Do Horse, middle and Cat with your hips. While carrying, do shoulder circling, Horse and Cat to the extent it is not disturbing your activity. After carrying, circle your shoulders backwards and move your hands in every possible direction, do Horse and Cat with your hips again.

If you do the lifting with your hand turned-out

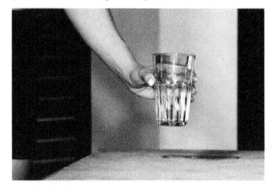

start doing it with your hand turned-in,

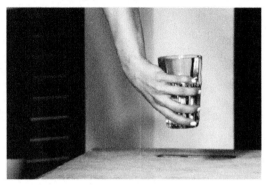

If you do the lifting with your hand turned-in,

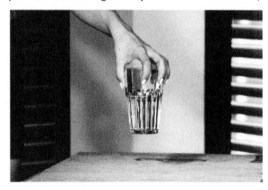

start doing it with your hand turned-out

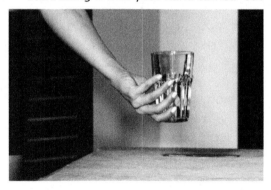

If you do the lifting or carrying with your elbow bent,
If you do the lifting with your shoulder up,

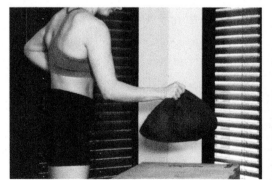

you need to start doing it with your elbow straight. bring your shoulder down; bring the shoulder backwards if it was forward.

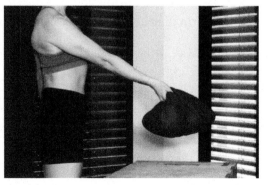

Lifting 9 liters of water

Consider the following example of lifting: you lift a sixpack of bottled water (9 liters) from the shopping shelf.

What am I doing?

I am lifting the water, carrying it and putting it down in the end.

Where is the weight resting?

The weight is resting on your feet and lower back. Before you lift, check that your ankles are in the middle, regardless of whether your feet are turned-out, -in, or parallel. You should not bring your hips to Cat or Horse, otherwise, with time, you will be at high risk of doing something wrong to your lower back, knees and ankles. This is because, in Cat or Horse, your lower abs (abdominals) do not support your lower back muscles.

Do Horse and Cat with the hips to find your Zero Position. With your back straight, bend your knees at least 30%, where 50% means the 90 degrees angle in your knees and your ankles (between your thigh and calf and between your calf and foot). Bend your arms, get your elbows close to your body, and grab the pack of water.[11] Press your hands towards each other while holding the pack, pull the water to your abdomen keeping the wrists in the middle.[12] Raise your upper body to a vertical position. Once your upper body is vertical, straighten your knees.

After you are done carrying water to your destination, do the reverse of lifting. Start with bending your knees, lean forward, and leave the water. Then roll up going through each bone in your spine (vertebra).

What is the exact opposite of the movement I am doing?

Use the same distance and the same angle in the opposite direction

Follow the opposite movements described above in the general "Liftin, carrying and putting something down". After lifting, do a stretch as described in the next paragraph.

Raise your arms to the sky. Hold there for a few seconds. If your wrist is turned-out when you are lifting, "point" the hand (or two) that you used. Press your back of hand with your other hand and straighten the elbow completely. Feel free to make fist with your hand while "pointing" it. Bring your hips to Cat (to relax the hip joint). If your wrist is turned-in when you are lifting, you have to stretch it with Flex rather than Point.

---

[11] While grabbing the water, do not lean forward more than 45 degrees with your upper body.
[12] Naturally, the water's trajectory will be diagonal rather than vertical in this case.

regardless of whether your feet are turned-out,

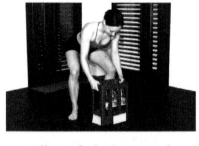 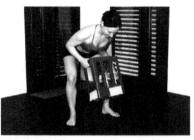 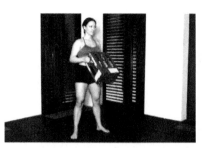

regardless of whether your feet are turned-in

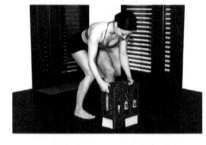 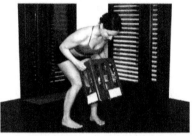 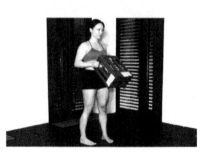

regardless of whether your feet are ,,, or parallel

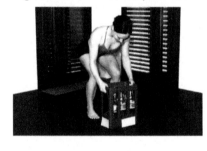 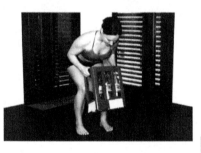 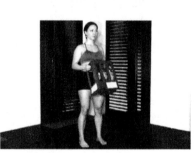

After you are done carrying water to your destination, ,do the reverse of lifting.
Start with bending your knees,

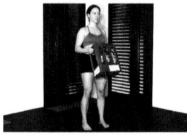 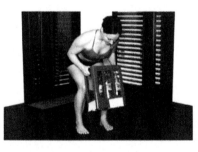 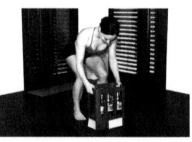

Raise your arms to the sky. If your wrist is turned-out when you are lifting, "point" the hand that you used.
Press your back of hand with your other hand and straighten the elbow completely

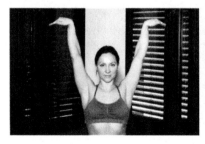 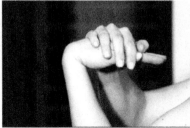 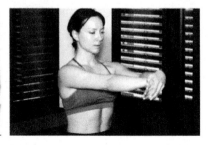

> **Flex**: A flexed hand is one where the wrist is actively pushing away from the body while the fingers pull towards the body.
> **Point**: Pointing is the opposite action of flexing. This means your palms should look inside of your forearm (make a "snake").

How do I improve?

The moment you start lifting something (even if it is a piece of paper), use the technique described in subsection "Sandwich". By doing this, you activate your core and stabilize the center of your body so that your lower back is not left to carry the weight alone.

Find different ways to lift.

For example, you can do Lunge with your left leg forward supporting yourself with your left hand on the left thigh. Straighten your back by bringing your hips to the middle, do not do Horse or Cat. Push your ribs down to activate your core, and lift the water. As an option, you can do the same with your right leg in the air.

Then stretch the muscles you have used: Stretch the arm using the same way as described in the opposite movement above. From standing, bring forwards your leg that was front in Lunge. Use Example 6 from section "Standing".

Wearing a backpack

When wearing a backpack, do not neglect the rubbing of the backpack against your back. With time, this may cause problems to your neck, shoulders, back, knees. To minimize this risk, follow Senda principles.

What am I doing?

I am wearing my backpack.

Flex   **Point**

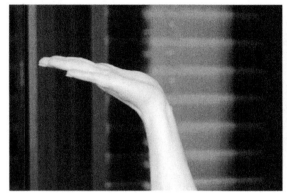   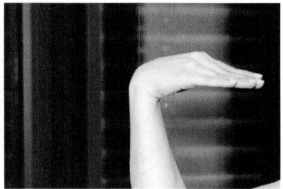

Find different ways to lift.   Then stretch the muscles you have used:

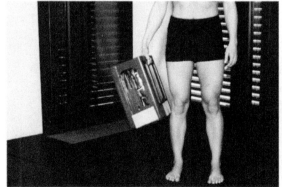   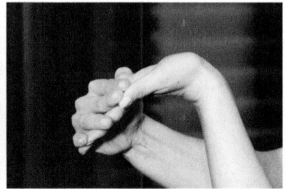

Where is the weight resting?

The weight is on the shoulders, middle back and lower back. If the weight is sufficiently great, it is likely to push your ankles, knees, hips and shoulders out of Zero Position. This is a natural reaction of your body to compensate the high load on the parts that are involved in wearing directly.

What is the exact opposite of the movement I am making?

Use the same distance and the same angle in the opposite direction

If your shoulders are in a forward position, bring them backwards, and vice versa. If one of the shoulders is raised, lower it. Do all this while still carrying the bag.

If your lower back is in Cat, bring it to Horse, and vice versa. If your back is tilted to the right, tilt it to the left, and vice versa.

Below we provide a few more detailed examples.

Example 1. If you walk doing a bit of Horse with your hips (this creates a "hole" between your lower back and the backpack), you need to do Cat with your hips.

Example 2. If you bring your shoulders to the front while wearing a backpack (your neck is leaning forwards, creating problems because of the big strain on the neck muscles) and have Cat in your hips while walking, bring the shoulders backwards and turn them out. Do Horse with your hips and bring your neck backwards.

Example 3. If your foot is turned out because your shoulder is brought backwards, you need to bring the shoulder forwards and turn your foot in at the same angle to the direction of your movement. Also check your ankle – roll it out in case it was rolled in.

How do I improve?

Make sure your ankles are in the middle. Feel free to choose the direction of your feet (parallel, turned-in, turned-out), but remember to keep switching.

Whenever you are wearing your backpack, use the "Sandwich technique" from time to time.

You need to

- minimize the friction of the back and the backpack
- stop wearing a backpack whenever you do not really need it
- find alternatives to wearing a backpack

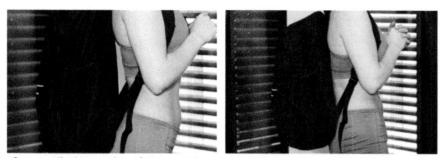

Example 1. If you walk doing a bit of Horse with your hips (this creates a "hole" between your lower back and....

Example 2.   If you bring your shoulders to the front while wearing a backpack ....

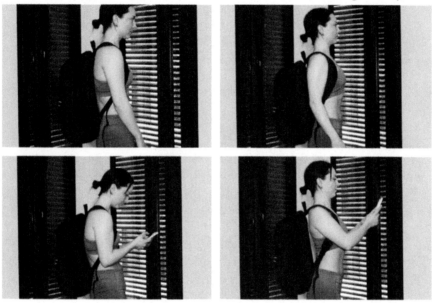

Example 3. If your foot is turned out because your shoulder is brought backwards,..

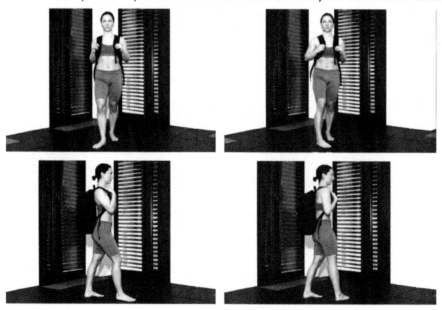

To minimize the friction, bring the straps of the backpack with your hands a bit closer to the neck. This will give your shoulders more freedom. You can also use a twist in your upper body. For example, twist to the left, walk for a while, then twist to the right, and walk for a while again.

Another option is to use one or both hands as a support for your backpack. Bring your hands behind your back and push the bag away from your back. Make sure there is no contact between your hands and your back.

Still another option is to grab the straps of the backpack with your hands around the level of your chest and pull them forwards. Then, pull the straps down slightly so that there are no "holes" between your back and your backpack left.

Whenever you do not really need to wear the backpack, do not wear it. Most obviously, put it off and drop it down whenever you are standing and waiting for something (even for a few seconds). Whenever you do so, circle backwards, first, only the shoulders, then the whole arms. This will keep the blood flow in the part of the body that was engaged in carrying the bag.

As an alternative to wearing a backpack on your back, you can wear it in front of you supporting it with one or both hands.

As another alternative, consider carrying the backpack in your hand for a while. Then use your other hand. Do not let the backpack touch your leg when carrying it in your hand.

You may also consider using all four different ways of carrying in turn: on your back, with your left hand, on your belly, with your right hand.

If you wear a backpack on both shoulders and you are not able to take it off, circle your shoulders a few times slowly from down to front to up to back. Move your hips between Horse and Cat, bring your hips to the left and to the right.

If you can take the backpack off from one shoulder, move the free shoulder the same way as described above or just find your own movement. If possible, circle your whole arm backwards as well. Do the same with the other shoulder.

Further examples to improve your backpack-wearing experience are:

Example 1. Find different places to put your purse and your phone. This way, the object (purse or phone) will not be pushing the same point on your body for too long. Explore different options: once you can put it in a side pocket, another time use the front pocket, and so on.

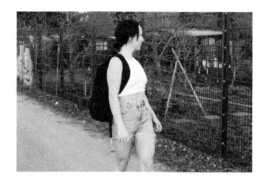

To minimize the friction, bring the straps of the backpack with your hands a bit closer to the neck. This will give your shoulders more freedom. You can also use a twist in your upper body. For example, twist to the left, walk for a while, then twist to the right, and walk for a while again.

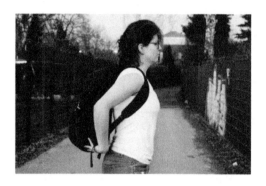

Another option is to use one or both hands as a support for your backpack. Bring your hands behind your back and push the bag away from your back. Make sure there is no contact between your hands and your back.

Still another option is to grab the straps of the backpack with your hands around the level of your chest and pull them forwards. Then, pull the straps down slightly so that there are no "holes" between your back and your backpack left.

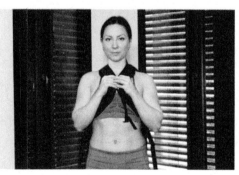
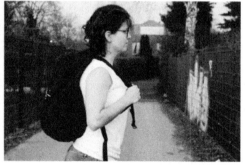

As an alternative to wearing a backpack on your back, you can wear it in front of you supporting it with one or both hands.

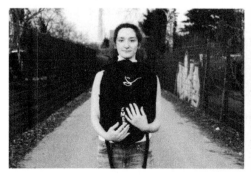
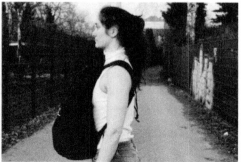

Example 2. Carry your backpack with your left hand. Bring your elbow as close to the left side of your body as possible. Bend your arm so that your forearm is at 90 degrees to your side and parallel to the floor. Rotate your forearm to the left without moving your elbow. Make sure you keep your shoulder and your wrist in the middle (check subsection Zero Position for shoulders and wrists).

Example 3. Carry your backpack on your head. Keep your neck in the middle.

Example 4. If you have to wait standing or sitting while having a backpack on you, bend your leg so that your thigh and shin form a 90 degrees angle. Put the bag over your bent leg. Feel free to use a wall, a friend, or another object as a support for your back if you feel unbalanced.

Example 5. Lift your arms together with your bag (unless it is too heavy for you to control), bring them up and to the back until you feel a stretch in your back. Do this every time after carrying your bag for a while.

Kids usually lean forwards because their bags are heavy for their lower back muscles. To counter the movement, they need to use the "Sandwich technique". They also need to keep ankles in the middle while walking as described above. And, of course, it is always better to prevent the problem rather than treat it – so make sure, as much as you can, that the responsible persons do not overload kids with books or any other stuff to put in their backpacks. If absolutely necessary to transport heavy stuff, please use a trolley-bag, regardless of your age.

Wearing a bag over your shoulder or in your hand

What am I doing?

I am wearing a bag over my shoulder or in my hand.

Where is the weight resting?

The weight of the bag is resting on one shoulder and the part of your body that the bag is touching (most likely your side).

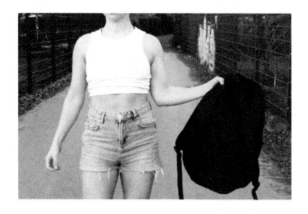

Example 2.   Carry your backpack with your left hand. Bring your elbow as close to the left side of your body as possible. Bend your arm so that your forearm is at 90 degrees to your side and parallel to the floor. Rotate your forearm to the left without moving your elbow. Make sure you keep your shoulder and your wrist in the middle (check subsection Zero Position for shoulders and wrists).

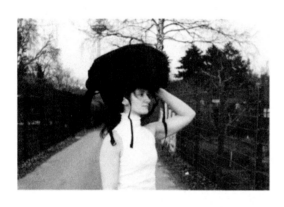

Example 3.   Carry your backpack on your head. Keep your neck in the middle.

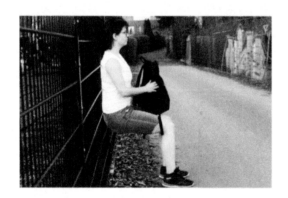

Example 4.   If you have to wait standing or sitting while having a backpack on you, bend your leg so that your thigh and shin form a 90 degrees angle. Put the bag over your bent leg. Feel free to use a wall, a friend, or another object as a support for your back if you feel unbalanced.

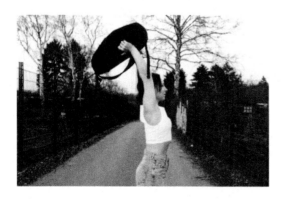

Example 5.   Lift your arms together with your bag (unless it is too heavy for you to control), bring them up and to the back until you feel a stretch in your back. Do this every time after carrying your bag for a while.

If you often keep the weight on one side of your body, it is likely to affect the way you walk. In particular, your foot on that side will most likely turn in.[13] The greater the weight of the bag is, the more likely it is to cause problems for you over time.

What is the exact opposite of the movement I am making?

Use the same distance and the same angle in the opposite direction

While still wearing your bag, do the opposite movement with your fingers, hand, elbow, or shoulder. Use the same techniques as described in the section "Lifting, carrying and putting something down". If your foot was turned in, turn it out by the exactly same angle to the direction of your movement, and vice versa. Next, if your foot was turned in, your ankle was probably rolled out, so you need to roll it in, and vice versa.

How do I improve?

Stop the contact of your bag with the part of the body it is rubbing, e.g., shoulder, hip, thigh, knee, shin. Use your hand to push your back away from your body. Switch between using your palm and the back of your hand to keep the bag away.

Find new ways to carry your bag with different parts of your body.

Example 1. Instead of having your bag hanging on your shoulder, you can put it on top of the shoulder and keep it there or slightly above, helping yourself with one hand.

Example 2. Carry the bag in your hand. Turn your hand out, carry the bag in this position for a while, then turn your hand in and stay in this position for a while.

Example 3. Lift the bag with both hands and bring it behind your neck, alternating between contact (touching) and no contact of your hands with your neck or your shoulders.

Example 4. Put the strap of the bag across your body, from the right shoulder to the left hip. Bring the left hand under the bag, grab the bag with your hand, and turn your hand out. Keep your elbow close to the side of your torso but do not let it touch your torso, and bring the hand back as far as you can. Make sure your shoulders are pushed back and downwards.

Example 5. Hold the bag with your hand with the arm straight and horizontal. Follow Zero Position for your wrist, elbow and shoulder; make sure to use the "Sandwich technique" with your core.

---

[13] If your foot is nevertheless turned out, which is rare, it is because your shoulder on which you carry the bag is brought backwards.

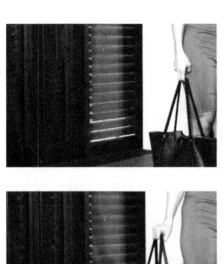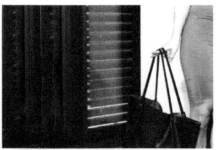

do the opposite movement with your fingers,

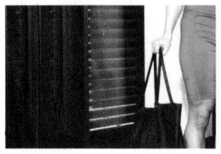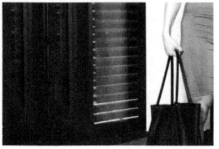

do the opposite movement with your , hand,

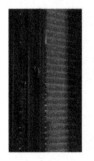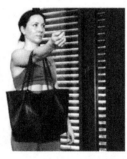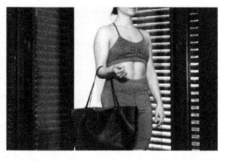

do the opposite movement with your , elbow,

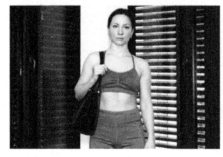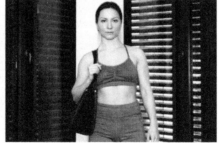

do the opposite movement with your .... or shoulder.

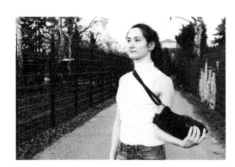

Example 4. Put the strap of the bag across your body, from the right shoulder to the left hip. Bring the left hand under the bag, grab the bag with your hand, and turn your hand out. Keep your elbow close to the side of your torso but do not let it touch your torso, and bring the hand back as far as you can. Make sure your shoulders are pushed back and downwards.

Carrying a child

Whenever you are carrying your child, use the "Sandwich technique".

What am I doing?

I am carrying a child.

Where is the weight resting?

The weight rests on your arm, shoulders, or neck.

What is the exact opposite of the movement I am making?

Use the same distance and the same angle in the opposite direction

Switch the position of your hips to the opposite from where they are. For example, if they are in Horse, move them to Cat; if they are left, move them to the right. Also, change the position of your neck to the opposite of where it is.

If you are carrying your child in one hand turned in, turn that hand (the wrist) out and keep it in that position for a while. Check your shoulders: refer to the technique used in the section "Lifting, carrying and putting something down".

If you are using a kangaroo to carry your child on your stomach or chest, move the shoulders to the opposite direction (e.g., if they are forward, bring them backwards), and minimize the weight on your chest and shoulders by lifting your child with your hands.

If you are carrying your child on one or both of your shoulders, just do the opposite to what you are doing to your shoulders. If the shoulders are raised, lower them; if they are in the front, pull them backwards.

Check your shoulders: refer to the technique used in the section "Lifting, carrying and putting something down".

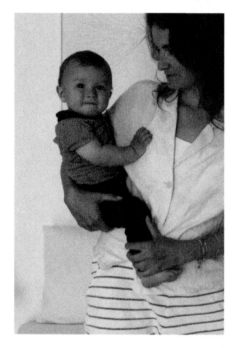 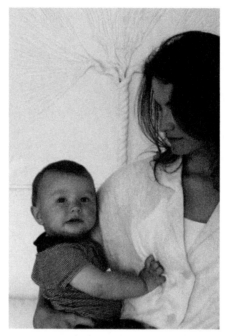

Check your shoulders: refer to the technique used in the section "Lifting, carrying and putting something down".

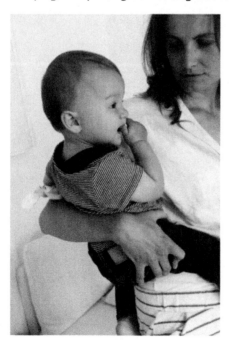 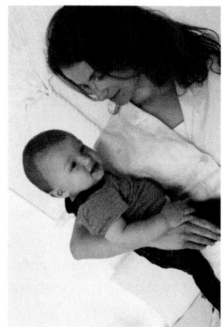

How do I improve?

Example 1. While carrying your child on one hand, turn the palm of that hand so that it faces the floor and bring your elbow higher towards your shoulder (but not all the way to the level of your shoulder). Use your second hand as a support.

Example 2. Carry the child with two hands and twist your upper body to the left and to the right. Hold in this position for a while. Use "Sandwich technique" while doing the twist.

Example 3. Make sure your legs are in Zero Position. If you are sitting or standing, open your legs more than hip-width and go into Second Position in dance (see the corresponding description in subsection "Sitting") with your feet turned out (make sure your ankles are in the middle). Hold your child close to your chest and push your knees outside (backwards) and back to where they were.

If you are using a kangaroo to carry your child on your stomach or chest, move the shoulders to the opposite direction (e.g., if they are forward, bring them backwards), and minimize the weight on your chest and shoulders by lifting your child with your hands.

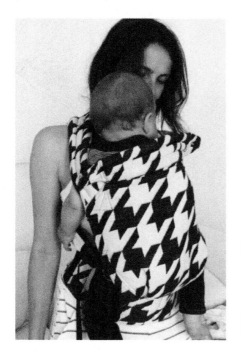 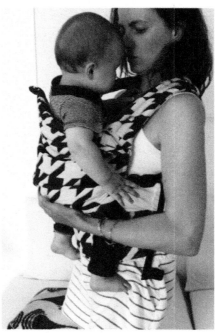

Example 2. Carry the child with two hands and twist your upper body to the left and to the right. Hold in this position for a while. Use Sandwich technique while doing the twist.

Example 3. Make sure your legs are in Zero Position. If you are sitting or standing, open your legs more than hip-width and go into Second Position in dance

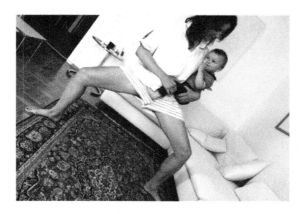 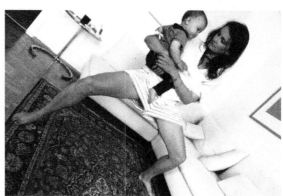

Remember,

Life is just a life

Note that if you are carrying something while walking up or down the stairs, you may want to first read the subsection "Lifting, Carrying and putting something down".

What am I doing?

I am walking stairs up. This can be just one step, e.g. stepping onto the bus, train or escalator.

Where is the weight resting?

The weight is resting on your feet, ankles, knees, and hips.

What is the exact opposite of the movement I am making?

Use the same distance and the same angle in the opposite direction

Refer to the principles described in the subsection "Walking" for doing the opposite movement to the one you are doing when Walking stairs up.

If you are walking stairs up with your ankle(s) rolled in, you need to start walking with your ankle(s) rolled out, and vice versa.

If you make your steps with only the front of your foot while the heel remains in the air below the level of the stair, you should start bringing your heel higher than the level of the stair.

How do I improve?

Make sure your steps are as soft as possible to protect your ankles, knees, hips, lower back, and neck. Bend your knee more than usual. Do this even when you step on the sidewalk or into the train/bus.

Example 1. Whenever possible, lift your feet higher than necessary.

Example 2. Take 2-3 stairs at a time. Raise your leg starting from the hip joint. Keep your ankles in the middle.

Example 3. Walk sideways on the stairs. Feel free to switch between feet parallel, turned out and turned in. Feel free to cross your legs or take steps with one foot always leading and the other following.

If you are walking stairs
up with your ankle(s)
rolled in,

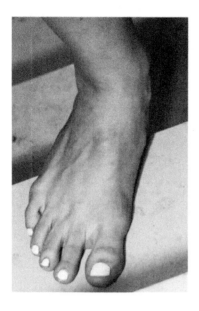
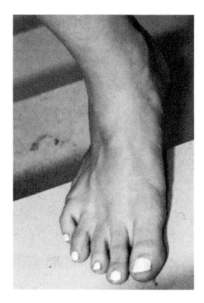

you need to start walking
with your ankle(s) rolled
out, and vice versa.

If you make your steps with only the front of
your foot while the heel remains in the air
below the level of the stair,

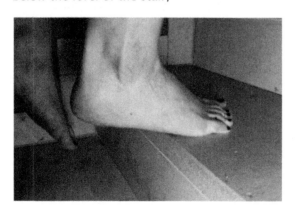
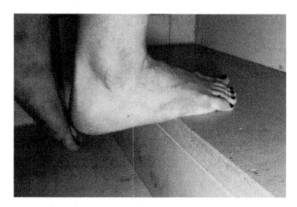

you should start bringing your heel higher
than the level of the stair.

Example 4. Challenge yourself to walk backwards on the stairs. For further challenge, get used to walking backwards without looking in the direction of your movement.

Example 5. Jump stairs up on both legs or on one leg only.

Example 6. If you want to use the staircase as a training device, put your foot two or three stairs higher than usual, make Lunge and stretch your other leg.

Example 7. Do the first step on the staircase. Note the level on which your knees are. Do the rest of the staircase at the same level, without going up or down (do not bounce). Feel free to switch between turn-out, parallel and turn-in with your feet. Make sure your ankles are always in the middle.

Example 8. If you are waiting on the escalator, stand on one leg and, bending your other knee, bring the foot of the other leg to your buttocks and keep your knees together. Feel free not use your hands to help your bent leg.

Example 9. Walk stairs up on your hands and feet (All Fours).

Walking down the stairs

What am I doing?

I am walking down the stairs. This can be just one stair when getting off a bus, train or escalator.

Where is the weight resting?

The weight is on your feet, ankles, knees, and hips.

What is the exact opposite of the movement I am making?

Use the same distance and the same angle in the opposite direction

Refer to the principles described in the subsection "Walking up the stairs" for doing the opposite movement to the one you are doing when walking down the stairs.

How do I improve?

Make sure your steps are as soft as possible to protect your ankles, knees, hips, lower back, and neck. Bend your knees more than usual. Do this even when you step out of the sidewalk or off the train/bus.

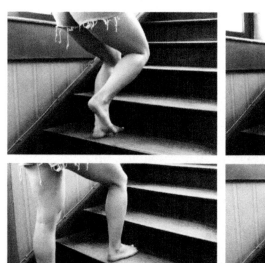
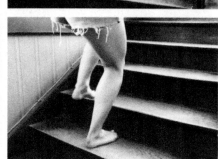
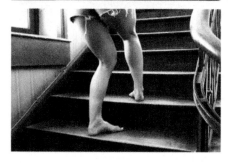
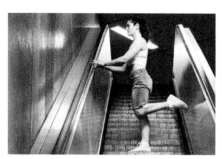
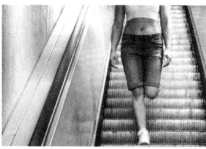
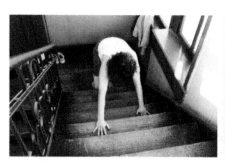

Example 7.
Do the first step on the staircase. Note the level on which your knees are. Do the rest of the staircase at the same level, without going up or down (do not bounce). Feel free to switch between turn-out, parallel and turn-in with your feet. Make sure your ankles are always in the middle.

Example 8.
If you are waiting on the escalator, stand on one leg and, bending your other knee, bring the foot of the other leg to your buttocks and keep your knees together. Feel free not use your hands to help your bent leg.

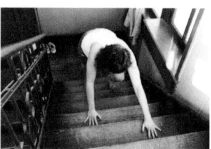

Example 9.
Walk stairs up on your hands and feet (All Fours).

119

If you walk down the stairs on your toes, it is likely that your knees are not bent enough, and that puts excessive stress on your ankles. You need to bend your leading knee more after every step in a flow. Your step should be soft and silent.

If you make your steps with the heel only while the toes remain in the air, you should start putting your whole foot on the stair. If there is not enough space to put your whole foot straight on the stair, put your feet turned-out.

Use the same examples as in the subsection "Walking up the stairs"

> Example 1. Keep your knees bent to Demi-plié and walk down the stairs with your feet parallel, turned-in/out, but keep your ankles in the middle.

> Example 2. Use wide steps and be soft with your foot to the ground.

> Example 3. If you are using the escalator, stretch your legs by using Example 6 from "Standing" section.

Running

What am I doing?

I am running. This includes running a few steps to catch a bus or train.

Where is the weight resting?

The weight is on your ankles, knees and hips. If you are also carrying something, the weight is also on your sides, shoulders and back.

What is the exact opposite of the movement I am making?

Use the same distance and the same angle in the opposite direction

Check the ankles, knees, as well as hips and follow the opposite movements described in subsection "Walking". If you are carrying something while running, also check the opposite movements described in subsections "Wearing a backpack", "Wearing a bag over your shoulder or in your hand", and "Lifting, carrying and putting something down"

How do I improve?

Move your jaws, neck, shoulders, arms and upper body as described in "Re-charging", steps from 2 to 7.

Walk on your toes during the day in order to strengthen your muscles (calves) and improve your speed.

Make sure your steps are as soft as possible and your ankles are in the middle to protect your ankles, knees, hips, lower back, and neck. If you need to roll your ankles in or out, do it slowly.

When running, use the "Sandwich technique". Keep the feeling as long as you can; then release your muscles for a while before engaging them again.

Example 1. Start running in "dahdaha", a slow running style: Run softly rolling your foot from your heel through the middle of your foot to your toes; then actively push your toes against the floor towards your next step. From time to time, exhale quickly twice on each step, then inhale long on two steps. You should produce a hissing sound while exhaling. Bend your arms and move your elbows slightly forwards and backwards while keeping them close to your body and arms bent.

Example 2. Run softly on your toes. Make sure your ankles are in the middle. Do this even if you are running only a few steps to catch a bus.

Example 3. Change the length of your step while running; change the rhythm; switch from toes to heels from time to time. Remember to run softly.

Example 4. Make large leaps at every step: lift your knee so high that your thigh is parallel to the ground; open your legs to facilitate a larger movement.

Example 5. Cross your legs while running (make crisscross steps).

Example 6. Challenge yourself to run backwards.

Example 7. Use the environment you are running in. For example, go up and down the stairs when you meet some, circle around a tree or a streetlamp, jump over a pit or a bench.

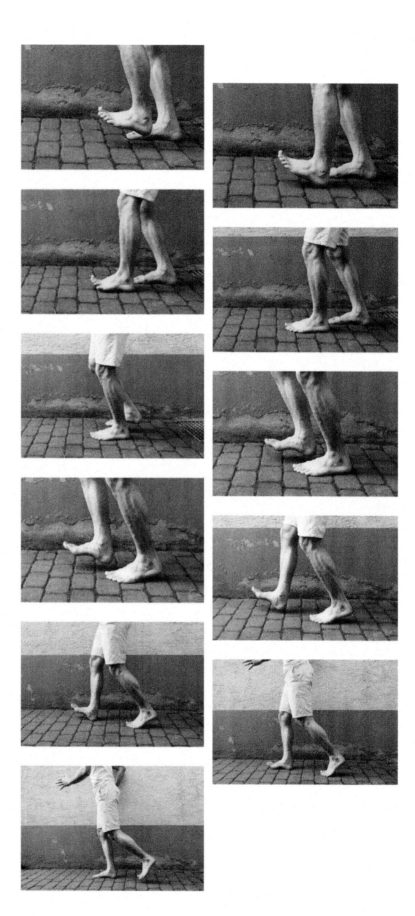

Example 1. in "Start running dahdaha",

What am I doing?

I am getting on or off a bike before or after riding it.

Where is the weight resting?

There are two ways to get on or off the bike.

First, if you swing your leg around the bike, the weight is on the hip, knee, ankle, and the foot of the leg that remains on the floor while you are getting on or off the bike.

Second, you may step directly over the pedal that is on the side of the bike next to you. In this case, the weight is on the hip, knee, ankle, and the foot that goes to the pedal first.

What is the exact opposite of the movement I am making?

Use the same distance and the same angle in the opposite direction

Check the ankle of the foot you are stepping on/off with. If your ankle is rolled in, roll it out, and vice versa. Do not worry about the opposite movement for the knee, because the knee will follow your ankle.

How do I improve?

Switch the leg you use for standing when getting on and off the bike – do your best not to repeat using the same leg more than twice in a row. This will help you to find new ways to get on and off the bike.

For further improvement, consider the following examples:

Example 1. Bend, more than usual, the knee of the leg you are standing on.

Example 2. Before getting on the bike, pretend getting on your bike by doing the same motion in the air, maybe slower, without actually getting on the bike (lift your leg, bend your knee, and hold few seconds). Repeat this movement 3-5 times (this will warm your hips up).

Example 3. Before getting on or off your bike, put your leg (it can be your calf, Achilles, or hamstring) on the saddle and stretch (lean forward with your upper body). Feel free to have your leg straight or slightly bent.

Example 4. Do Example 6 from section "Standing" before and after riding a bike.

If
your
ankle
is
rolled
in,

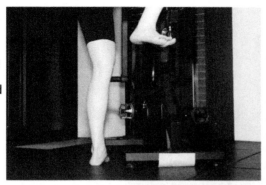 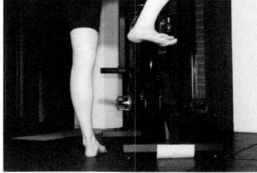

roll
it
out,

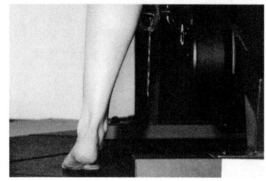 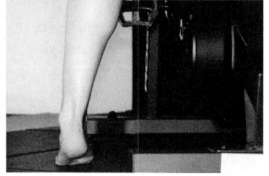

If your ankle is rolled in,   roll it out,

Example 3. Before getting on or off your bike, put your leg (it can be your calf, Achilles, or hamstring) on the saddle and stretch (lean forward with your upper body). Feel free to have your leg straight or slightly bent.

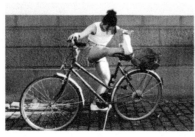 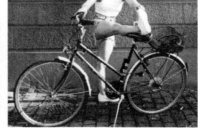

Example 5. To get off your bike, push your bike forwards with two hands, push your hips backwards (this will likely make your upper body bend forwards).

Example 6. Getting off your bike, cross your legs. You will need to bend your knees more than usual while landing.

Example 7. While getting off the bike on the right side, raise your left leg to the left as high as you can while keeping it straight, circle with it backwards before putting it on the floor.

Example 8. Start with the same movement as in Example 6 but circle your straight leg from the left to front before landing. You will need to balance the bike by switching the hold of your hands on the handlebar.

Riding a bike

What am I doing?

I am riding a bike.

Where is the weight resting?

The weight is on the feet, ankles, knees, hips and on the lower back. Depending on the riding style, a significant part of the weight can be on your hands.

What is the exact opposite of the movement I am making?

Use the same distance and the same angle in the opposite direction

Check your ankles: If the ankles are rolled in, roll them out, and vice versa. Pay attention to your hips: Bring them to Cat if they are in Horse and vice versa.

Check each leg. In case the distance between your knees is larger than the distance between your feet, bring the knees closer together, and vice versa.[14] If you are riding with your foot turned out, you need to turn it in and vice versa.

Check your hands. In case your wrists are turned in, turn them out and vice versa.

Check your shoulders.[15] Bring them backwards if they are forward; bring them down if they are up.

---

[14] Note that Zero position for the knees when you are biking is at the same distance between them as between the feet.

[15] When your body needs to relieve the pain in your lower back, it lifts your shoulders.

Example 7.

Example 8.

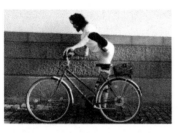 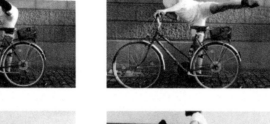 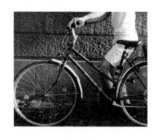

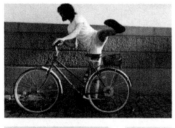 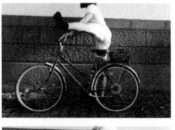 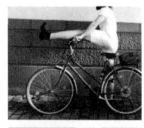

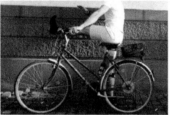 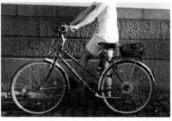 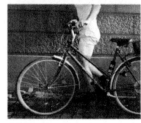

turn them out

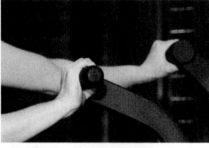 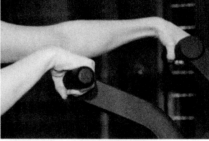

Check your hands. In case your wrists are turned in,

Cat

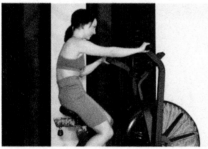 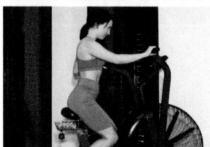

Pay attention to your hips: Bring them to ... if they are in Horse

bring the knees closer together

you need to turn it in

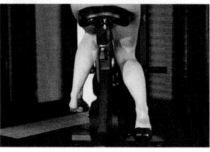 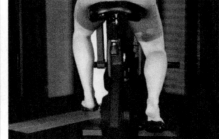

knees is larger than the distance between your feet,

your foot turned out,

How do I improve?

Move your neck, shoulders, arms and upper body as described in "Re-charging", steps from 2 to 7.

Whenever you are riding a bike, use the "Sandwich technique". Do this as long as you can; then release your muscles for a while before engaging them again.

Keep your hips moving between left, Cat, right, Horse and middle while driving, but hold in each position for a while.

If you are carrying your backpack while riding, follow the techniques described in the examples in subsection "Wearing a backpack".

> Example 1. Keep the distance between your knees the same as the distance between your feet while riding. Make sure your ankles are in the middle. Feel free to use toes or heels for pushing the pedals.

> Example 2. Use a bike saddle that cushions the stress of the riding. Lift your hips away from the saddle as often as possible.

> Example 3. Starting from Zero Position for the Neck, turn your head left and right, up and down to warm up your neck. Whenever you pass a hindrance with your bike (a groove or a bump), bring your neck back to Zero position to be prepared for the stress to your vertebrae caused by the hindrance. Also lift your hips from your bike saddle.

> Example 4. Alternate between pushing the pedals with your heels (your foot is Flex), your middle foot, and your toes (your foot is in Relevé).

> Example 5. Challenge yourself to ride with one leg only. You are free to put the other leg on the bike or leave it in the air. Remember to be fair; for example, if you make 20 rotations with your left leg, make another 20 with your right leg.[16]

> Example 6. Ride with your legs turned out (hips, knees, feet) and push the pedals with the heels. Make sure to keep your ankles in the middle.

Riding a scooter

What am I doing?

I am getting on a scooter; I am riding a scooter; or I am getting off a scooter.

---

[16] If one of your legs is stronger than the other, use the weaker leg more until your legs get balanced.

128

Where is the weight resting?

The weight is on your feet, ankles, knees, hips, hands, and neck.

What is the exact opposite of the movement I am making?

Use the same distance and the same angle in the opposite direction

If your foot is turned in, turn it out, and vice versa. For other opposite movements, refer to the techniques described in the subsections "Getting on/off the bike" and "Riding a bike".

If your scooter is not electric and you are using your left leg more than the right one (to propel the scooter), start using the right leg more (it is probably your weaker leg), and vice versa.

How do I improve?

Move your neck, shoulders, arms and upper body as described in "Re-charging", steps from 2 to 7. Use the "Sandwich technique" from time to time.

Example 1. Be soft when getting on and off by bending your knees more than usual.

Example 2. Ride with your left leg forward and turn your left foot out. Also turn your right foot out. Bring your ankles to the middle and keep them there. Bend your knees slightly to accommodate all the grooves and pebbles you are meeting on the way. In case you are bored, bend your knees more – you will feel how smooth your ride is becoming.

Example 3. Use examples from "Riding a bike" section.

Getting in/out of a vehicle

What am I doing?

I am getting in or out of a vehicle before or after I drive it.

Where is the weight resting?

The weight is on the foot that is stepping in or out of the vehicle. The part of your weight is also on the hip on the side that you are using for stepping in or out.

Depending on the vehicle and the way you are getting in/out of it, your weight could also be on your ankles and knees and on your hands and forearms.

What is the exact opposite of the movement I am making?

Use the same distance and the same angle in the opposite direction

Check the ankle of the leg you are stepping in/out with. If it is rolled in, roll it out, and vice versa. If your hand and forearm are turned in, turn them out and vice versa. Pay attention to your hips and bring them to Cat or Horse depending on your position, as described in subsection "Walking", Example 2.

How do I improve?

Find different ways to get in and out of a vehicle. Always getting in/out of a vehicle in the same way leads to knees, hips, or back injuries.

    Example 1. Alternate which leg you use to get in/out of the vehicle.

    Example 2. Step backwards, sit down, and then pull your legs.

    Example 3. Use both legs together when getting out of the vehicle. Follow Example 1 to Example 5 from subsection "Sitting" that refer to changing the way you stand up from sitting.

Driving a vehicle

What am I doing?

I am driving a vehicle.

Where is the weight resting?

The weight is on the ankles, hips and lower back. The weight could also be on a side of your body or on your elbow.

What is the exact opposite of the movement I am making?

Use the same distance and the same angle in the opposite direction

If you are driving with your upper body straight and two hands on the steering wheel, do the opposite of what your lower back does: because you are probably in Cat, do Horse.

If your shoulders are raised and forward, pull them backwards and down. Your neck may be leaning forward, bring it back (while keeping your eyes on the road).

Suppose your weight is on the right side of your body (or your right arm, right elbow). Your right shoulder is likely forward and raised – pull it backwards and down. Continue pushing with your ribs to your left side and push with your elbow to get your chest higher up to the left. Do Horse with your hips as you probably are in Cat. Bring your neck left if it was leaned to the right.

In case your weight is on the left side while you are driving, use the same technique as described in the paragraph above.

If you step on the gas, brake or clutch pedal with your foot turned out, you need to start pushing it with your foot turned in and vice versa. Pay attention to your ankles and roll them in or out if necessary (see Section "Standing" for pictures).

How do I improve?

Move your neck, shoulders, arms and upper body as described in "Re-charging", steps from 2 to 7.

Keep your hips moving between left, Cat, right, Horse and middle while driving, but hold in each position for a while. Put a soft pillow behind your lower back to prevent your hips and lower back from doing too much Cat. Follow all the possible examples from subsection "Sitting" and use the examples below.

> Example 1. Lift your leg whenever possible and make Flex and Point with your foot a few times. Circle your foot Heartwise (see section "Standing", Heartwise box). Make sure that you reach the maximum diameter of your circle.

> Example 2. If your car has automatic transmission, lift your free leg up and put it back down. Repeat a few times. Do the same with manual transmission whenever you get the chance.

> Example 3. Find a way to straighten your leg to feel stretch around your knee for few seconds.

> Example 4. Pretend you want to slap someone behind your back. You make a twist with your upper body, stretch your arm behind, and come back.

> Example 5. In case you are stuck in a traffic jam (only when your car is not moving), pretend you want to pick up something from the floor and put it beside you. Do the knee stretch from Example 3 longer. If it is possible, bring your knee to your chest and hug it for a few seconds.

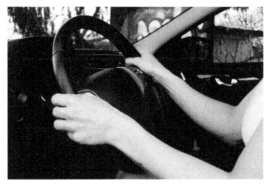 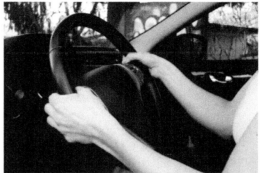

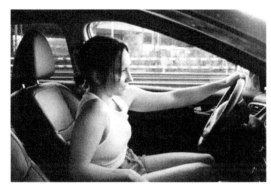 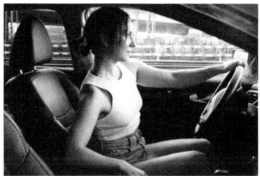

Suppose your weight is on the right side of your body (or your right arm, right elbow). Your right shoulder is likely forward and raised – pull it backwards and down. Continue pushing with your ribs to your left side and push with your elbow to get your chest higher up to the left. Do Horse with your hips as you probably are in Cat. Bring your neck left if it was leaned to the right.

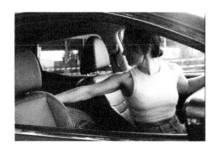

Example 4. Pretend you want to slap someone behind your back. You make a twist with your upper body, stretch your arm behind, and come back.

Your dream is

your Imagination – live your

dream in your

daily life until

you reach your goal

What am I doing?

I am lying down.

Where is the weight resting?

Where your weight is depends on how you are lying. If you are lying on your back, the weight is on your neck, shoulders and hips. If you are lying on your side, the weight is on your shoulder, your hip, your knee, and your ankle. If you are lying on your stomach, the weight is on one side of your neck, on your shoulders, your chest, your hips, as well as the knee and the ankle of the leg that is turned out/in.

What is the exact opposite of the movement I am making?

Use the same distance and the same angle in the opposite direction

If you usually use a pillow under your head, move this pillow down and put it under your upper body and neck, so that your head softly falls back. Hold this position for a while till your body tells it is enough.

If your hips are in Cat, bring them to Horse.

If your mattress is so soft that the hips are sinking into it (below an imaginary line from head to the feet), put a pillow under your buttocks towards your thighs. The idea is to lift your hips above the level of the head and feet, your body forming a concave arch.

How do I improve?

Do a stretch before you sleep to relax the muscles you used and to tell your body it's time to sleep. If you do not stretch the parts of your body that you used during the day, your body will do the stretch, but at the minimum level. It is not fair to use your body for 15 hours a day or more and then to give it few hours for unconscious stretch during your sleep. Even if you had an opportunity to sleep for 15 hours a day, it would still not be enough for your body to recover as it needs a focused stretch. Be fair to your body and it will be fair to you by not giving you illness or pain.

If you usually use a pillow under your head,

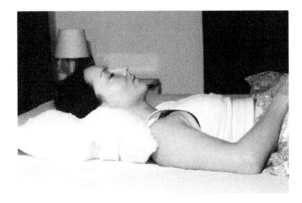 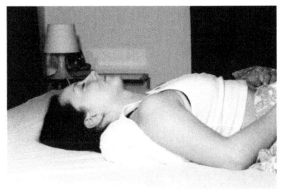

move this pillow down and put it under your upper body and neck

If your mattress is so soft that the hips are sinking into it

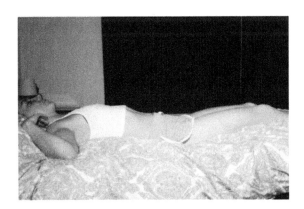 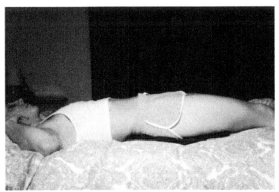

put a pillow under your buttocks towards your thighs.

Example 1. If you are lying on your side, put pillows between your feet and between your knees (to reach your hip-width); put your cheek on your arm, using a thin pillow between your cheek and your arm. Also put a pillow under your waist (side).

The pillow under your head should be thin enough to keep your neck straight; the feet and knees pillows should be of the same size and thicker than the pillow under your head.

Example 2. If you often wake up with pain in your lower back, you should sleep with a pillow under your buttocks so that your body forms a straight line.

Example 3. In case you sleep on your stomach, put a pillow under your stomach and hips, until you are in slight Cat with your hips.

Example 1.

If you are lying on your side, put pillows between your feet and between your knees (to reach your hip–width);

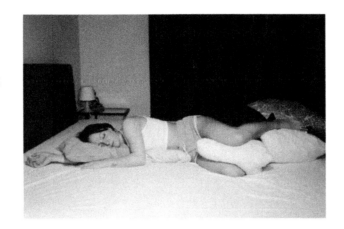

Example 2.

If you often wake up with pain in your lower back, you should sleep with a pillow under your buttocks so that your body forms a straight line.

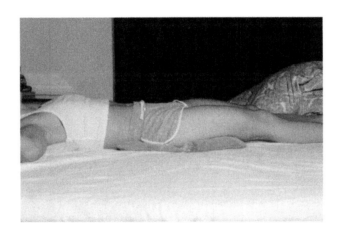

Example 3.

In case you sleep on your stomach, put a pillow under your stomach and hips, until you are in slight Cat with your hips.

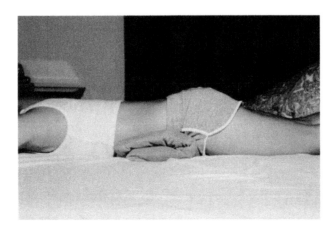

Conclusion

Let us now repeat the main take-home messages of this book again.

For every movement you do repeatedly throughout your day, you need to do the opposite movement – in the best case, right after you did the original one. If it is possible to break a complicated movement in parts, do the opposite after each part of the original movement.

Furthermore, for the movements that you are doing regularly for a prolonged period (weeks, months, years), you need to start exercising the opposite movements regularly until you bring your body back into balance. This can take weeks, months, or even years, depending on how often you repeat the opposite movement and how long you have been exercising the original movement.

Throughout the first part of the book, you have learnt to do the movements that are the opposite to what you normally do. That is a good starting point, but you should by no means stop here. To keep functional the body parts in use, you need to pay more attention to them. During the whole day, you need to move your joints in all possible directions considering the joint movement and not your possible directions! You also need to do warm-ups for the parts of your body which are going to be used in your activity.

Use the routine described in "Re-charging" as many times as you need throughout your day. If your activity involves many repetitions of the same daily routine, do not be shy to repeat the examples for improvement as many times as your body needs.

Do not get discouraged if you cannot master all the examples described in this book: It is sufficient to carry out a few. Also, do not try to do too many exercises one after the other. Quality always comes before quantity: Make sure you do a few examples properly; then, after a while, you can switch to the next, more challenging example. The most important is to find your own creative movements. Always discover new ways to improve yourself!

Your energy level is changing all the time. It is different from morning to evening; it depends on your mood and on your nutrition. Therefore, you need to take care and pay attention to your every movement especially when you are tired (most injuries happen when you are tired).

Do not justify your laziness or fear with the lack of consistently gathered empirical evidence of the effects of Senda on human body. Your lifestyle, the way you make your usual movements, brings you to the point when you notice, sooner or later, that something went wrong. Senda cannot make it worse, because all it proposes is to listen to your body and do what it needs: First, by doing the opposite movements to undo the damage; then, by releasing your creativity to improve the resilience to unexpected movements. Senda can only make things better for you because it never asks you to make the movements that do not suit you. That is why there is no need to wait for the results of a controlled experiment that would compare two groups of similar individuals, members of one practicing Senda and of another not practicing it as required for pharmaceutical drugs. Senda is no drug; it has no negative side effects – you just need to think about yourself differently and give your own body a chance!

In the end,

Senda is doing sports without doing sports,

it is moving without moving.

Extra pictures

waking up

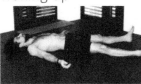 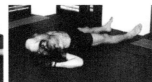 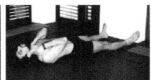

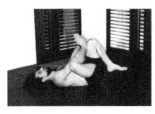 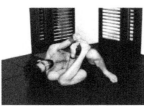

Then, do a little warm-up that consists of small movements, starting with toes, ankles, slowly going to knees, hips, back, shoulders, elbows, wrists, fingers, mouth, eyes, and, finally, neck.

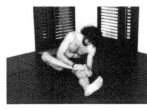 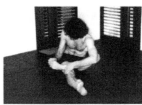 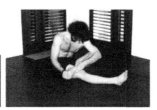

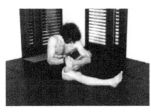 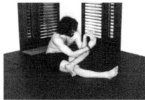 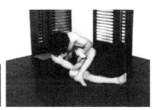

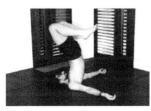 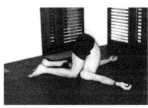

If you do not stretch the parts of your body which you are going to use during your day, the body will not be well-prepared to the challenges of the day.

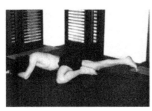 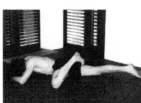 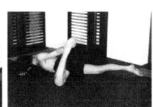 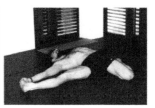

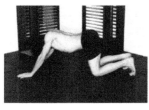 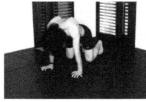

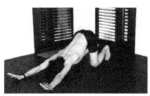 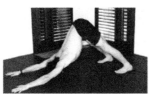 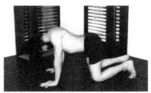

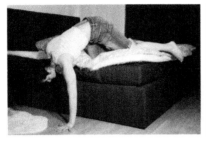 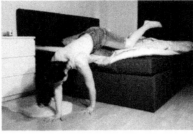 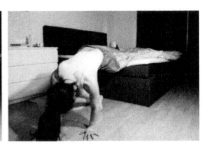

Example 2. If you are lying on your back, you have three options to change your position before standing up: (1) turn to your left side, (2) turn to your right side, or (3) turn around to your stomach. Choose a body part you want to stand on first: This could be hands,

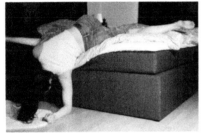 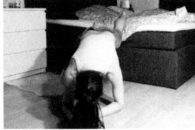 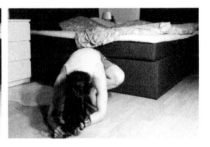

elbows,

knees.

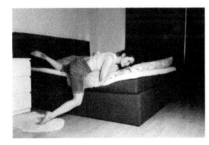 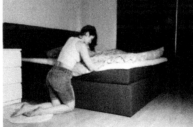 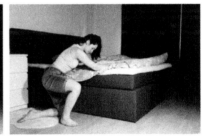

For example, go into a handstand to get out of your bed.

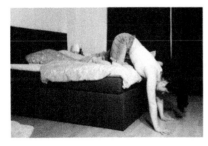 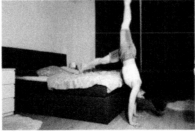 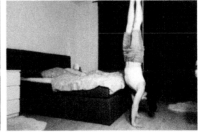

Feel free to alternate this warm up with two modifications:

1– Follow the steps till and including 8. while standing on one leg or switching the legs from one...

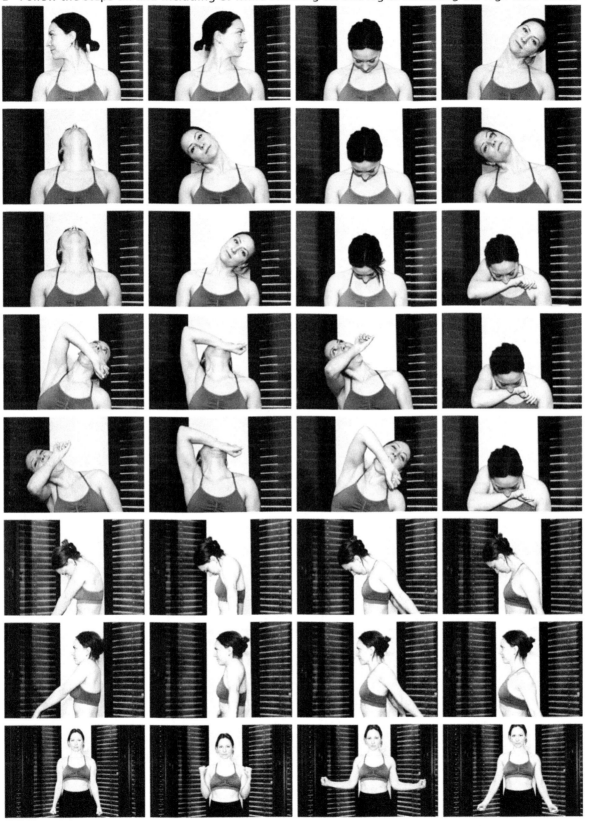

Example 1– Follow the steps till and including 8. while standing on one leg or switching the legs from one to another. From step 9. on, do everything normally.

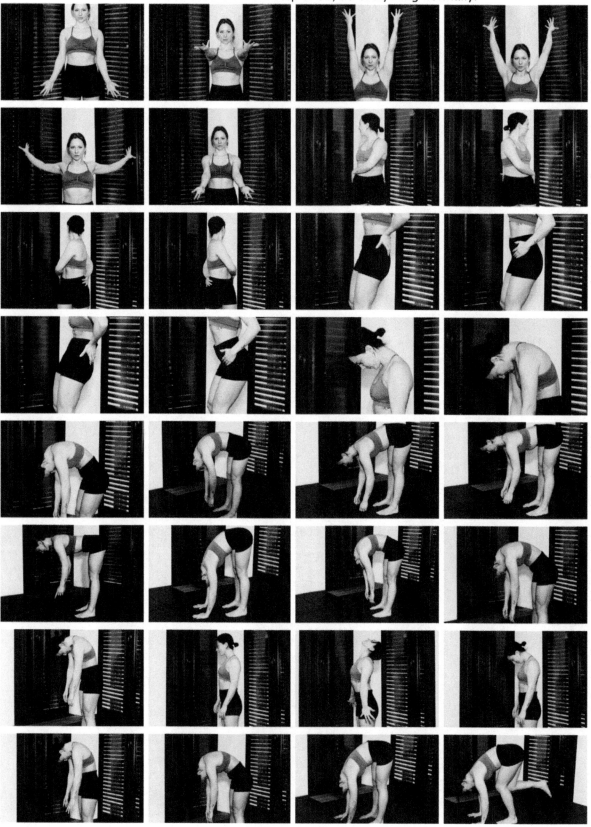

151

Example 1– Follow the steps till and including 8. while standing on one leg or switching the legs from one to another. From step 9. on, do everything normally.

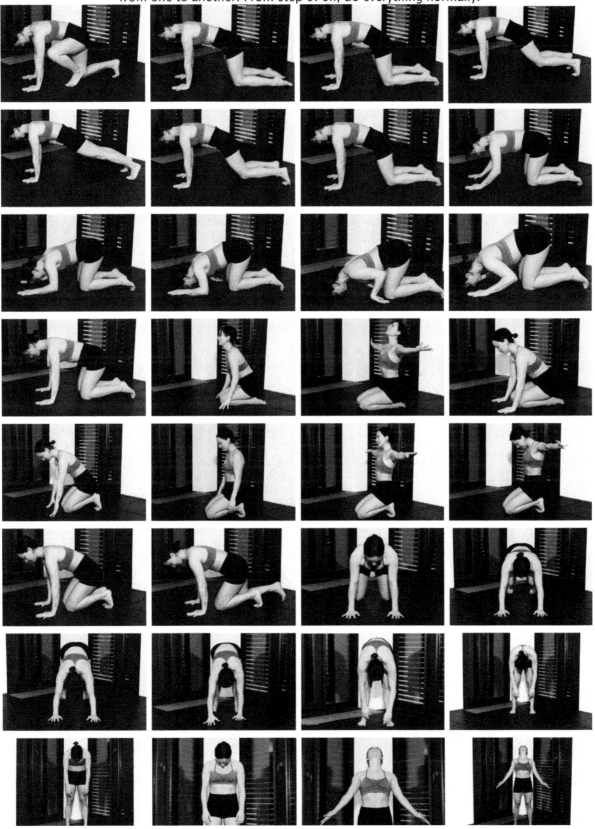

Example 2– Do the steps till and including 11. with your back on the floor to find new positions of pain to work on. From step 12. on, do everything normally. At the end, do step 16. on your back.

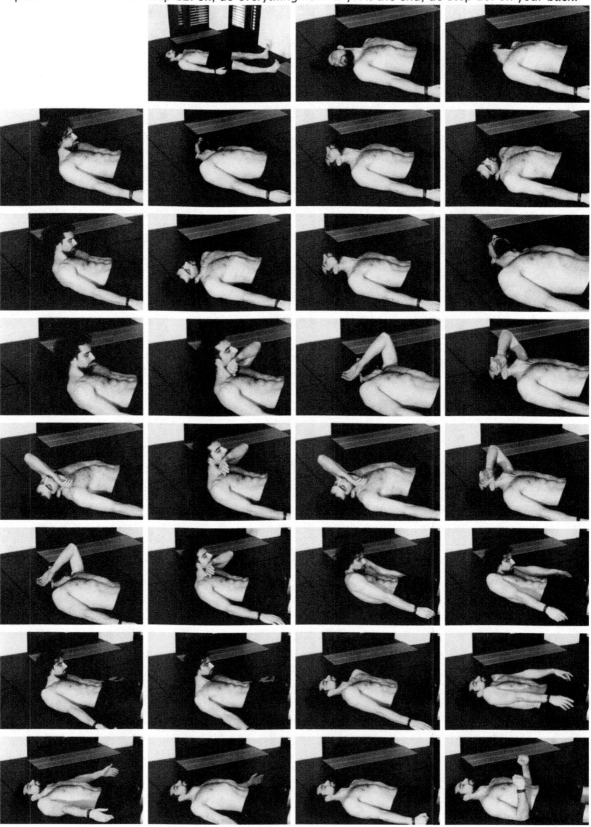

153

Example 2– Do the steps till and including 11. with your back on the floor to find new positions of pain to work on. From step 12. on, do everything normally. At the end, do step 16. on your back.

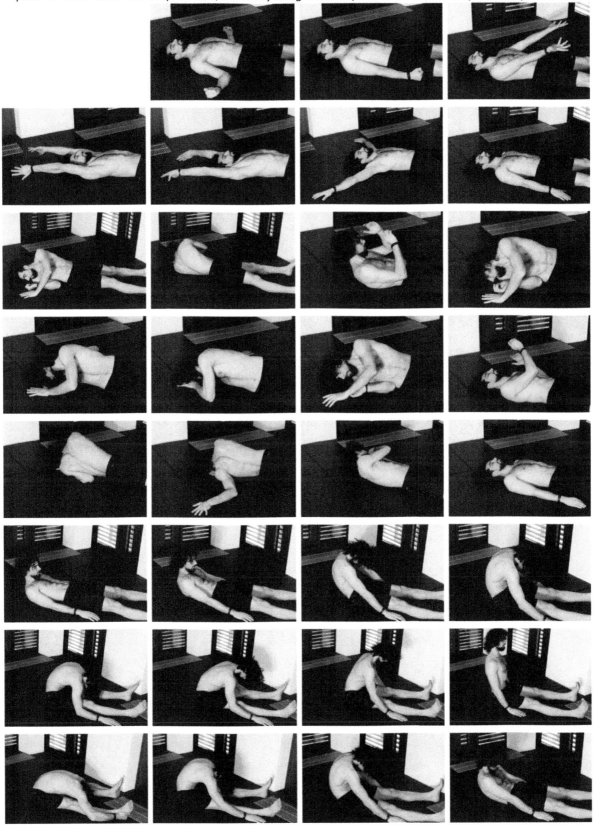

Example 2- Do the steps till and including 11. with your back on the floor to find new positions of pain to work on. From step 12. on, do everything normally. At the end, do step 16. on your back.

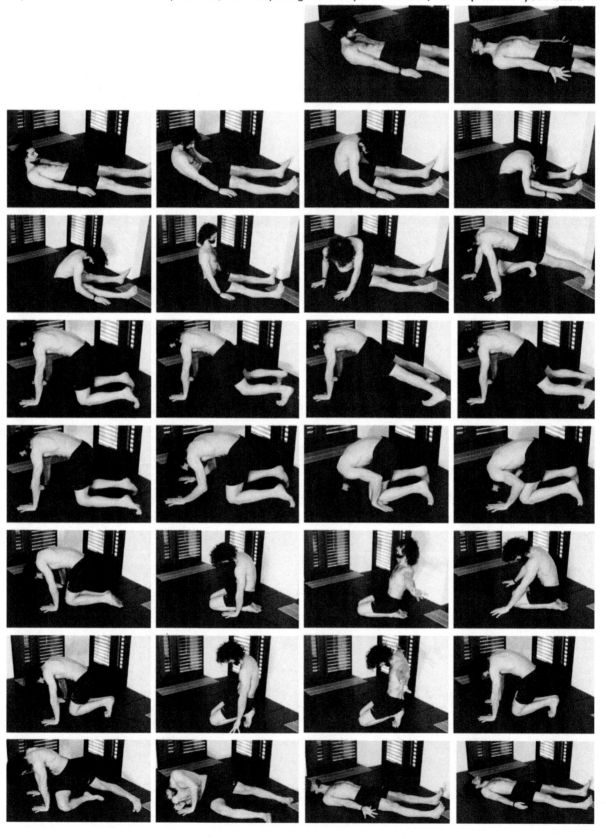

155

Example 1.   Circle your feet in the same direction slowly. Make a couple of circles, first starting left-upwards, then in the opposite direction.

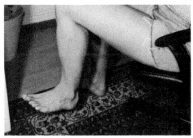 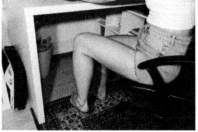 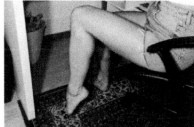

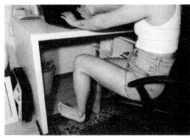

Example 2.   Move your hips in a circle while also shifting your weight. Start from left, then do Horse, then right, then Cat – then do it all over again a few times.

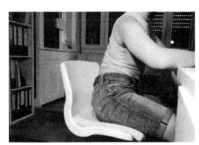 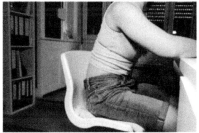 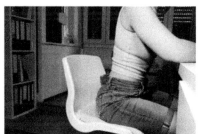

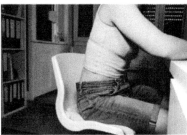

Example 3.   If you are sitting and writing for a prolonged time (for work or for studying), put your elbows on a support (do not let them "hang in the air" freely/unsupported) and lean with your upper body forward. Otherwise, you may get problems with your wrists, arms, shoulders, or neck.

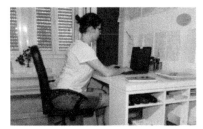

Example 7. While sitting, bring your feet to hip-width (see Hips) and raise your heels. Turn your feet in so that your knees touch each other. Stay in this position for a few moments.

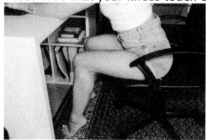 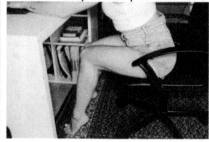 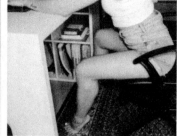

Example 8. While sitting, bring your feet and knees together. Without moving your upper body, bring your legs to the left in a twist - hold few seconds, then do the right side.

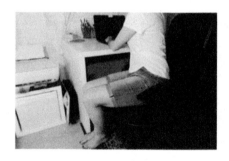

Example 10. Pretend your pen has fallen down and stand up to pick it up. Next, move your hips a few times.

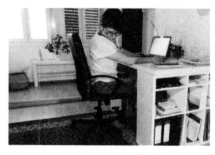 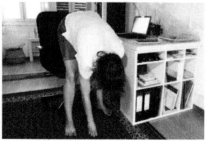

Example 15.
When you are putting your make-up on, follow the techniques described in the examples above. Challenge yourself to use the hand you are not normally using while putting the make-up on.

Make sure there is enough light in the room not to strain your eyes.

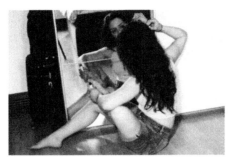
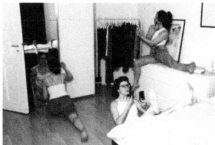
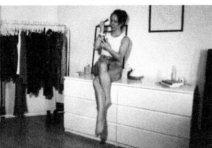
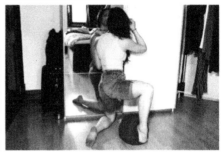

Example 16.
While doing your hair, circle your shoulders backwards. Use any of the examples above while doing your hair whenever possible.

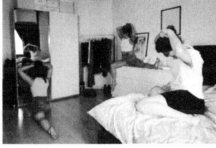
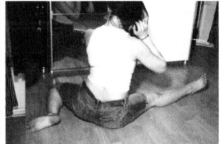
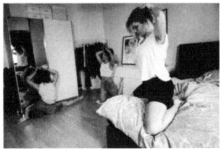
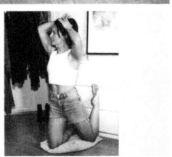

Example 18.
Challenge yourself to put your seat aside and do a squat ("sit in the air") on one or both legs. Follow the Zero Position principles for your big toes and ankles.

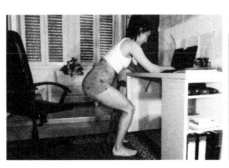
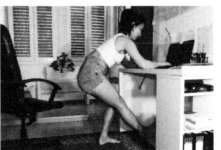

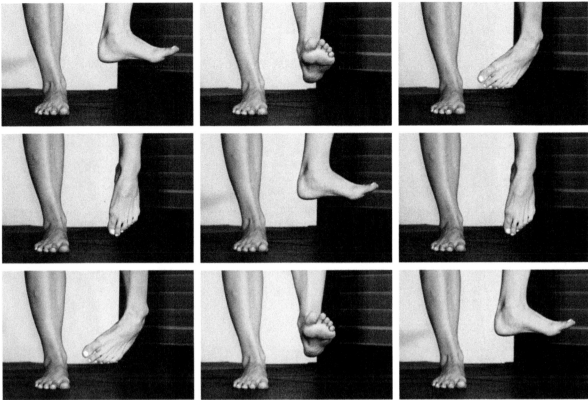

Example 1. Rotate your free foot, first Anti-heartwise, and then Heartwise. Pay attention to keep the ankle of the standing leg in the middle.

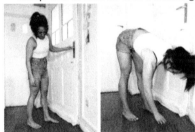

Example 4. Pretend something has fallen down – pick it up keeping your legs straight. Reach with your hands to the floor as much as you can. If you already can put your palms on the floor, do not stop there. Hold for a few seconds and then roll your upper body up as in step 10 of "Re-charging".

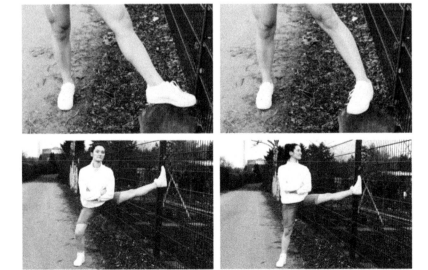

Example 5. Find an object to put your left foot on, in front of you. Do not put too much weight on your left knee by leaning over it. Keep your heel on its place and start moving your left foot slowly and carefully to the left and to the right. Pay attention to your ankles – keep your ankles in the middle! You should feel some tension in your left thigh and in your left hip.

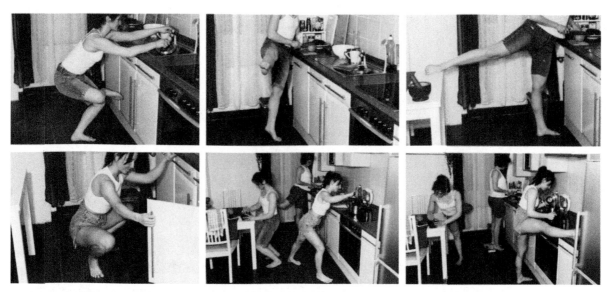

Example 12.   While you are standing and cooking, do the exercises described above and Sandwich technique.

Example 13.   When you are putting your make-up on, follow the techniques described in the examples above. Challenge yourself to use the hand you are not normally using while putting the make-up on.

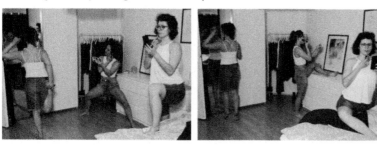

Example 14.   While doing your hair, circle your shoulders backwards. Use any of the examples above while doing your hair whenever possible.

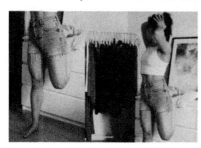 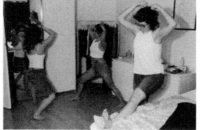

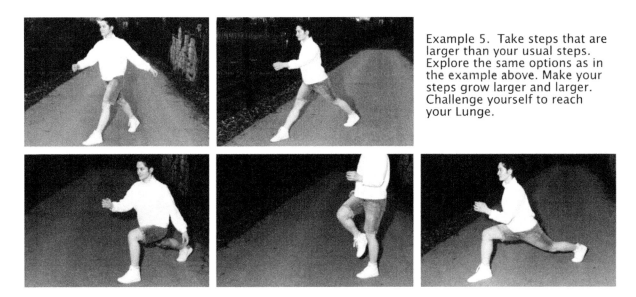

Example 5. Take steps that are larger than your usual steps. Explore the same options as in the example above. Make your steps grow larger and larger. Challenge yourself to reach your Lunge.

Example 7. Walk sideward crisscrossing your legs. Play with the distance: Take smaller and larger steps, change your leading leg. Change direction, experiment!

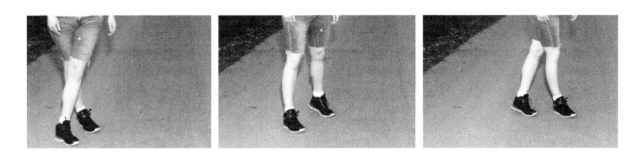

Example 11. When you are cleaning, use your weaker hand for a couple of days or months until it becomes as strong as the stronger hand. Then, start alternating your hands and use them equally.

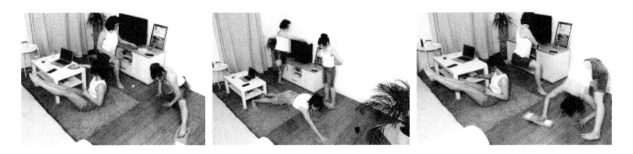

Example 1. Instead of having your bag hanging on your shoulder, you can put it on top of the shoulder and keep it there or slightly above, helping yourself with one hand.

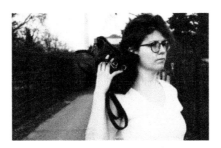

Example 2. Carry the bag in your hand. Turn your hand out, carry the bag in this position for a while, then turn your hand in and stay in this position for a while.

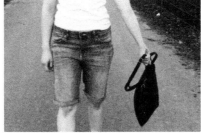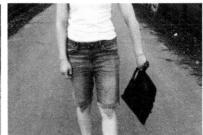

Example 3. Lift the bag with both hands and bring it behind your neck, alternating between contact (touching) and no contact of your hands with your neck or your shoulders.

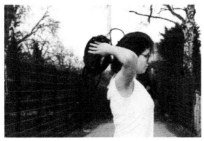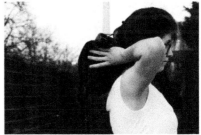

Example 5. Hold the bag with your hand with the arm straight and horizontal. Follow Zero Position for your wrist, elbow and shoulder; make sure to use the Sandwich technique with your core.

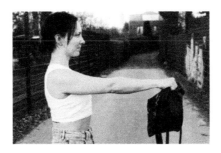

Example 3. Walk sideways on the stairs. Feel free to switch between feet parallel, turned out and turned in. Feel free to cross your legs or take steps

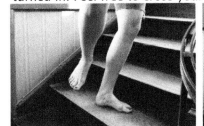 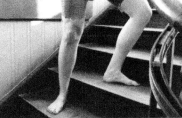 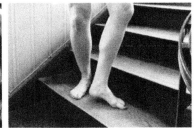

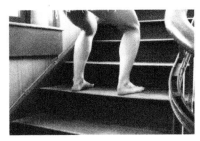 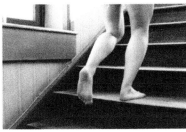

Example 5. Jump stairs up on both legs or on one leg only.

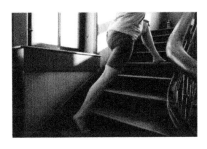

Example 6. If you want to use the staircase as a training device, put your foot two or three stairs higher than usual, make Lunge and stretch your other leg.

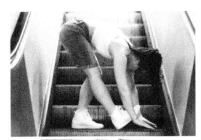 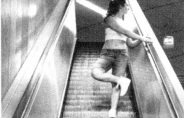 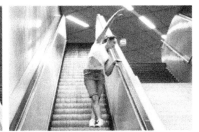

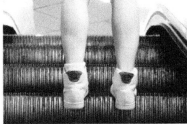 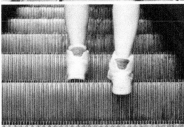

Example 8. If you are waiting on the escalator, stand on one leg and, bending your other knee, bring the foot of the other leg to your buttocks and keep your knees together. Feel free not use your hands to help your bent leg.

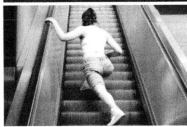 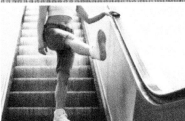 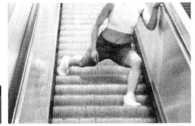

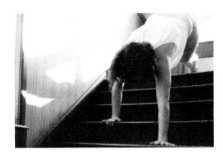

Walk stairs down on your hands and feet (All Fours).

Example 1.   Keep your knees bent to Demi-plié and walk down the stairs with your feet parallel, turned-in/out, but keep your ankles in the middle.

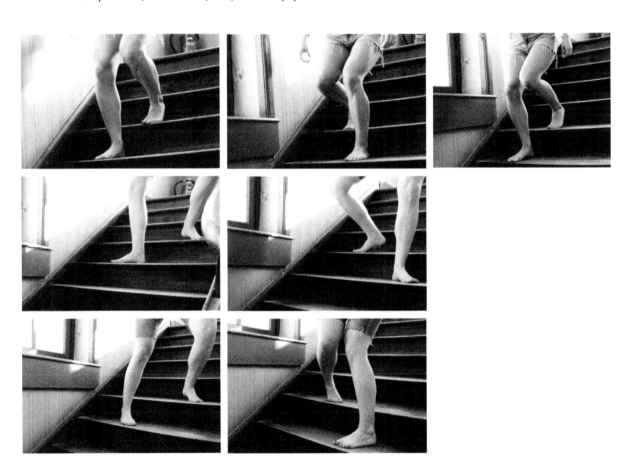

Example 1. Start running in "dahdaha", a slow running style: Run softly rolling your foot from your heel through the middle of your foot to your toes; then actively push your toes against the floor towards your next step. From time to time, exhale quickly twice on each step, then inhale long on two steps. You should produce a hissing sound while exhaling. Bend your arms and move your elbows slightly forwards and backwards while keeping them close to your body and arms bent.

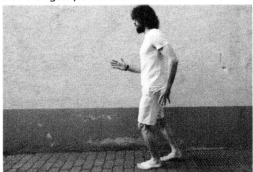

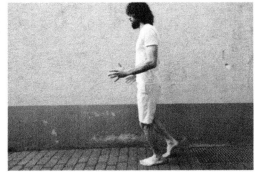

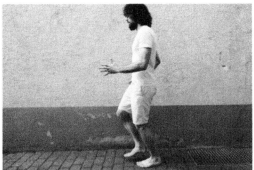

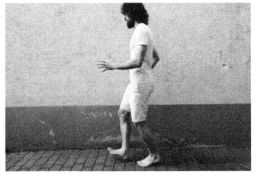

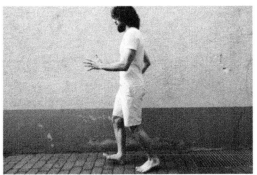

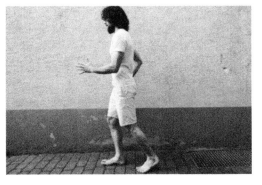

Example 2.

Before getting on the bike, pretend getting on your bike by doing the same motion in the air, maybe slower, without actually getting on the bike (lift your leg, bend your knee, and hold few seconds).
Repeat this movement 3–5 times (this will warm your hips up).

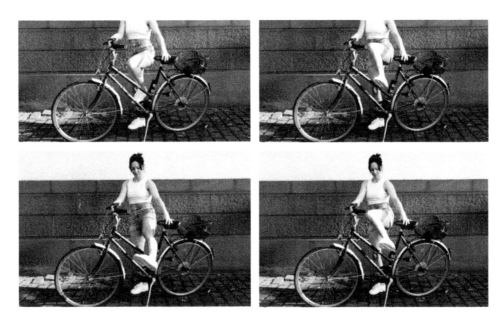

Example 5.

To get off yor bike, push your bike forwards with two hands, push your hips backwards (this will likely make your upper body bend forwards).

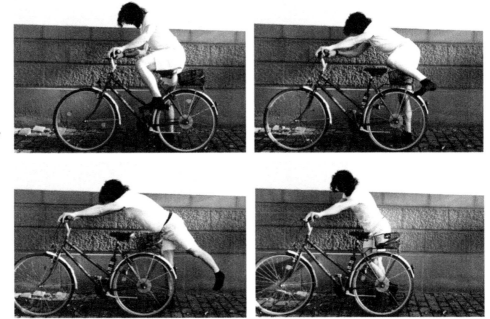

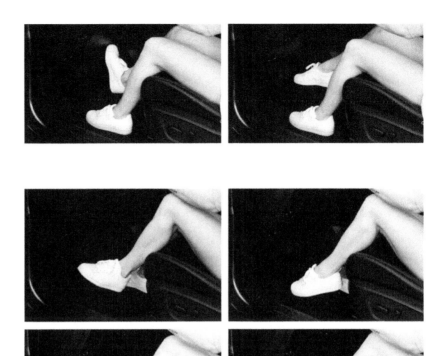

Example 1. Lift your leg whenever possible and make Flex and Point with your foot a few times. Circle your foot Heartwise (see section Standing, Heartwise box). Make sure that you reach the maximum diameter of your circle.

Example 3. Find a way to straighten your leg to feel stretch around your knee for few seconds.

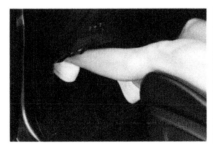
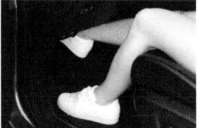

Example 5. In case you are stuck in a traffic jam (only when your car is not moving), pretend you want to pick up something from the floor and put it beside you.

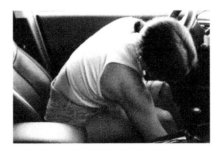

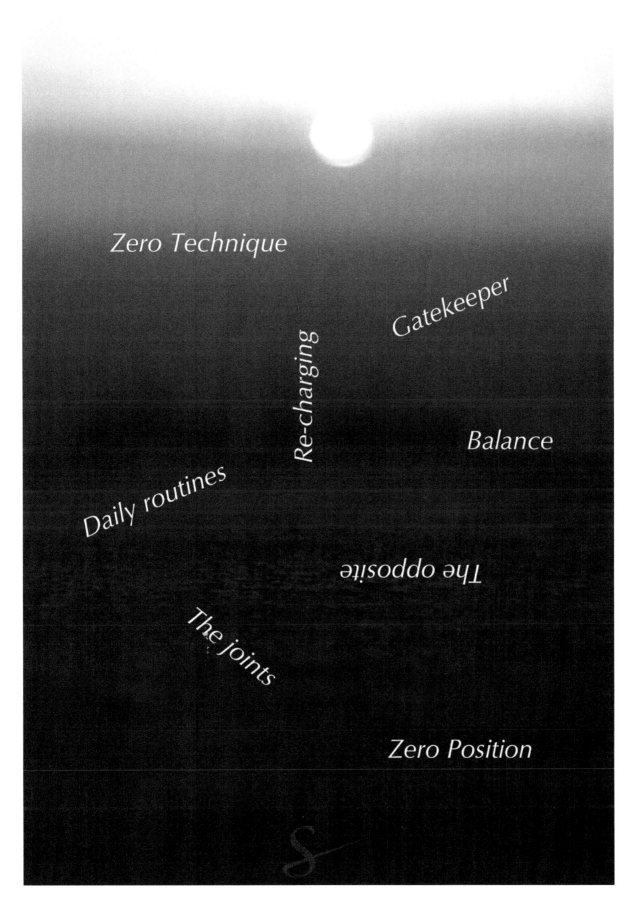

Zero Technique

Gatekeeper

Re-charging

Balance

Daily routines

The opposite

The joints

Zero Position

Time is what limits you!
Free yourself from time

Basics of lifestyle

Before/after food

Before/after eating, stand up and stretch your body (like a tiger), especially your stomach. This is what some of animals do before/after eating – stretching like a tiger/cat is the way to tell your body that the food should go to each part of your body. Open your mouth to the maximum – you can use your wrist as a help – to stretch your jaws. Put your tongue out to the maximum and move it in all possible directions. Moving the joints in all possible directions (considering the joint movement and not your possible directions) is the only way to make sure they get enough nutrients to stay functional.

Brush your teeth

After food or drink, stand up, rinse your mouth and then brush your teeth (use water only) without touching your gums.

Floss your teeth

Floss your teeth twice a day. This should not happen less than one hour after food.

Drinking water

Drink your water in a comfortable sitting position – this will protect your stomach from subsidence caused by water falling into it. When you are sitting comfortably, the water falls on the walls of your stomach calmly and gently. The idea is not to let stomach hanging so that it moves down when water comes into it. When you are sitting, the internal organs hold each other so that your stomach is fixed in its place. If you have to stand while drinking, use "Sandwich technique" to protect your stomach from subsiding.

Stomach pain

When you have pain in your stomach after eating something wrong or more than enough, lay down on your left side for a while, then turn to the right side and lie again for a while.

Helping blood circulation

Lie down on your back and straighten your legs. Put 1-3 pillows (or any other object) under your heels to raise the legs about 20-25 cm up.[17] Hold this position for 1-2 minutes. This is especially recommendable before going to sleep and after waking up.

---

[17] When you lift your legs not higher than about 25 cm, your blood flows in your body without putting too much strain on your heart.

Before/after food

stretch your body (like a tiger), especially your stomach – stretching like a tiger/cat is the way to tell your body that the food should go to each part of your body. Open your mouth to the maximum – you can use your wrist as a help – to stretch your jaws. Put your tongue out to the maximum and move it in all possible directions. Moving the joints in all possible directions (considering the joint movement and not your possible directions) is the only way to make sure they get enough nutrients to stay functional.

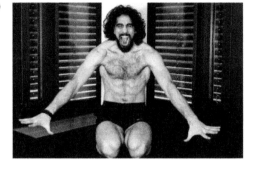

Here are few examples:

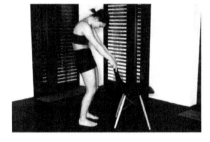 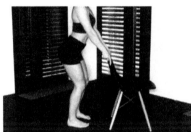 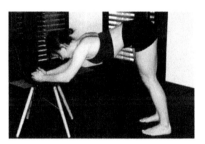

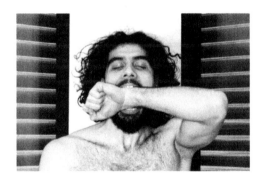  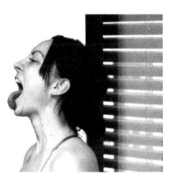

Helping blood circulation

Lie down on your back and straighten your legs. Put 1–3 pillows (or any other object) under your heels to raise the legs about 20–25 cm up. Hold this position for 1–2 minutes. This is especially recommendable before going to sleep and after waking up.

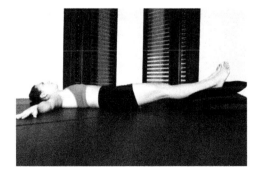

Free your feet

Take off your shoes and socks whenever possible, move the joints in your feet (use your hands to push and pull your toes) and let your feet breathe for as long as possible. This is especially recommended while you are sitting and as a break from walking.

Massage your feet along the lines from toes to ankles and further up every night. This will help your nervous and lymphatic systems to better perform their functions.

Free your toes

Put a long sock over and under your toes (like a snake or a wave) – start under the big toe then over the second toe, under the third toe, over the fourth toe and under the small toe. Lifting the middle toe gives the toes the position opposite to which they usually find themselves in. This is especially recommended while you are sitting and walking at home.

> For example, put a hair tie around your big toes and spread your feet to the point where the hair tie is a bit stretched. Start moving the toes apart, then back to each other without moving your feet. Repeat a few times. This is a competition between your big toes and it should not involve movements of the other parts of your foot. This exercise is important to prevent degenerative development in your big toes, often triggered by wearing tight shoes/socks or high heels.

Take care of your voice

Do not drink anything warm after running or any other activity that heats you up (e.g., singing or dancing), otherwise your immune system gets weaker and your voice will become hoarse later.

Keep yourself warm

When it is cold outside, you should cover your joints with warm clothes. Wear long socks to cover your ankles and the area above them.[18] Do this even if you do not feel cold in the cold weather.

Wear windproof pants (and other windproof clothes if possible) to protect your knees. Also cover your lower back to protect your kidneys. Do not let your feelings deceive you, wear protective clothing whenever it is cold (windy, rainy, snowy) outside even if you do not feel cold.

---

[18] This is necessary to make sure your knees, hips and internal organs in hips area stay healthy.

Free your toes

Put a long sock over and under your toes (like a snake or a wave) – start under the big toe then over the second toe, under the third toe, over the fourth toe and under the small toe. Lifting the middle toe gives the toes the position opposite to which they usually find themselves in. This is especially recommended while you are sitting and walking at home.

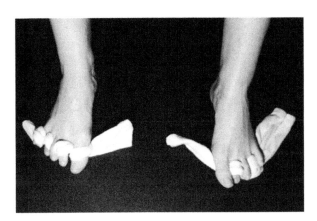

For example, put a hair tie around your big toes and spread your feet to the point where the hair tie is a bit stretched. Start moving the toes apart, then back to each other without moving your feet. Repeat a few times. This is a competition between your big toes and it should not involve movements of the other parts of your foot. This exercise is important to prevent degenerative development in your big toes, often triggered by wearing tight shoes/socks or high heels.

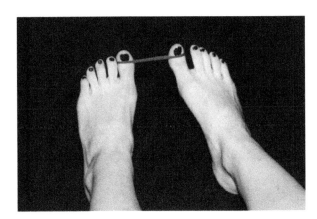

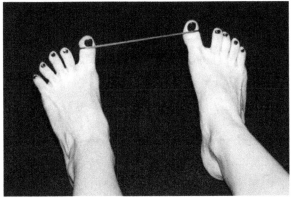

Be nice to your nose

Cover your nose and mouth when it is cold outside to keep the temperature of your body constant. This is especially important when you step into a warm place from a cold outside, and vice versa. Put something warm (e.g., bottle of water) on your nose when your nose gets cold or when you start to get sick and your nose starts to drop mucus.

Charge your brain

Lay your forehead and nose softly on the floor; the backs of your hands are facing the floor with the fingers pointing to your feet. Hold for a while. Do it as often as you can during your day. This is important for your brain to have enough blood supply to prevent neurological diseases.

Deserve the water you drink

To put 2-3 liters of water you drink a day to a good use, you need to move and sweat (even if sweating is minimal). This way, your kidneys will use this water to clean your body.

Keep your spine flexible

It will help you and everyone around you (especially those who are 18 and younger) to be aware of the following. The last part of the column (sacral curve) has 9 vertebrae, 5 of which get fused together in sacrum and 4 of which get fused together in coccyx. The fusion may be completed at the age between 18 and 30. However, if you practice any sport which improves the flexibility of your hips and the lowest part of your backbone (sacral curve), the 9 vertebrae will remain flexible.

Special flexibility moves for your lower back and hips will not allow the 9 vertebrae of your sacral curve to get fused if you do these moves every day. In case the vertebrae got fused already by the time you are reading this book, start moving your lower back and hips in all directions more than you have to. Do the special flexibility movements for your lower back and hips in order to make the vertebrae unfused again.

For example, you can do the gymnastic bridge exercise or downward-facing dog. Another example is to do extreme Horse while walking and use 2-3 pillows behind the lower back while sitting, to also reach extreme Horse. Do each example long enough to feel it.

Deserve the food you eat

Eat very slowly, enjoy your food, do not mix many kinds of food at the same time. It takes 4 minutes for the kidneys to clean the blood of the whole body. When you are eating or drinking fast, your kidneys do not have a chance to clean all the toxins that come into your blood stream with the food and drink. When you are eating or drinking slowly, give your kidneys enough time to clean the toxins and therefore protect your other organs from them.

Empty your stress

Change your position immediately when one of the following happens:

- you get any news which you do not like;

- you are arguing;

- something at work drives you crazy.

If you do not change your position, the stress will produce fat in the body. When you are getting stressed out, the adrenal gland secretes Cortisol hormone. When this hormone stays high and is not used by moving the body, it causes:

a) your immune system to perform below its potential;

b) stiffness in your muscles, especially around the parts of the body that are used;

c) fat to be deposited in the upper body (from the lower belly till the shoulders and neck).

The solution is: change your position. If you are sitting, start walking and vice versa. If you are lying down, stand up and vice versa. The best is to burn that stress out, keep moving till you empty that feeling (e.g., go to box sack, do crunches and pushups).

You can't help if you don't improve

and you don't improve until

you start helping

By keeping the whole channels (blood vessels) clean and flexible in your body, you can protect your body from illness, injury or pain. You can also help your body heal and get rid of pain.

This part of the book is to help you understand what your body needs and to know what to do when you have pain, even if it is in one of your internal organs. So, if you have pain, injury, or illness, do this part of the book as a first step and the first part of the book as a second step.

Zero Position and Zero Technique are just the base for the whole knowledge about the body. Zero Technique is working on the Roads, Bridges and, ultimately, Gatekeepers to release the damage in the body.

Zero Technique is not enough to come to an end of the story with your pain; you will need to change your whole lifestyle (think, wake up, move, eat, go to sleep).

I think of the body as a beautiful town that has the following elements:

The Castle is your organs.

The Gatekeepers are your jaws, neck, shoulders, and hips.

The Bridges are your elbows and knees.

The Roads are your wrists, ankles, fingers, and toes.

The Gatekeepers

The Gatekeepers have a double mission:

1. They protect your organs. When you let one of the 4 Gatekeepers neglected, you weaken the protection of your organs.

2. They warn you. When one of your organs has a problem because of your nutrition habit, one of your Gatekeepers will become inflexible.

There is no one who can survive without the Gatekeepers. Pay attention to your Gatekeepers and keep them healthy. The mission of the Gatekeepers is to protect the Castle (organs). In order to keep your Castle functional, you should start moving all your 4 Gatekeepers more than you have to.

For example: If you stop moving your hips in all possible directions while sitting or standing, it will cause problems in your organs around the hip area. And if you do not move your neck, jaws or shoulders more than you have to, this will affect your organs around your jaws, neck and shoulders.

If you are missing your foot/hand or your leg/arm, then work on the corresponding Gatekeeper (hip or shoulder). If you have no arms or legs, do not stop moving. Walk on your stumps by moving your hips and use your shoulders more than you have to.

Free the joints and muscles of pain immediately after you start feeling it by working on the Roads (joints) in your foot or hand, then by working on the Bridges (knees, elbows) and, finally, by working on the Gatekeepers: neck (atlantoaxial joint), jaw, shoulder, and hip.

You may ask yourself, why do I not work on the Gatekeeper directly? It is correct to work on the Gatekeeper directly if you have no arm(s) or leg(s) because there are no channels from the toes to your hips or channels from the fingers to your neck. But if you have these channels, they should first be cleaned by working on the Roads and Bridges before you can start working on the Gatekeepers.

The moment you start to move and work on the joints: jaws, neck, shoulders, hips, feet or hands – you will immediately start releasing the damaged part of your body from pain.

There are 2 reasons why the Gatekeepers send you pain signals when they are damaged: (1) misusing them, and (2) unbalanced food.

1. When you use one of your Gatekeepers in a limited way every day, it starts to get neglected or overused, and also unable to reach some positions. This unbalanced Gatekeeper will not be able to let the blood flow smoothly in and out of your Castle anymore. The lack of proper blood circulation makes you get those pain signals to balance your movements and free your Gatekeeper.

   Before starting to affect your organs, the Gatekeeper will give you a lot of warning signals. First, these will be stiff muscles in a specific area of the Gatekeeper. Then, you will feel the pain in the bridge or middle back. If you do not fix the damage, it will go to the Roads or lower back. Next, the pain will appear in your Gatekeeper. Finally, if you continue ignoring all the warnings, the damage will come to your Castle (organs). To prevent this, you have to be moving the Gatekeepers in all directions to keep them functional.

2. The food story starts with questions. When do you start drinking/eating something? What are you drinking/eating during your day? Is it the right food for your body? Do you always feel good after drinking or eating? When do you take your last drink/meal before going to sleep?

Every drink or meal enters your body and, if it does not harm any of your organs, it is the correct food for you.

Make sure you follow these 3 rules with your food:

Rule one: Keep your food balanced between alkaline and acidic.

Rule two: Do not eat the same food and do not drink the same drinks next day.

Rule three: Do not repeat eating acidic food every day.
Alkaline food is mostly what comes from the ground and acidic food is processed food and mostly is not coming from the ground.

After getting correct food, your body will experience the following: Feeling light, getting energy, no gases in your colon, no pain in your stomach, no bad mood, strong immune system, no extra weight. If you get correct food regularly, you will also defecate (go to the toilet) every day.

The stomach renews itself each 3-5 days. So, if you had a kind of food that bothers you, stop eating it for at least five days, and then try it again.

When the organs are getting problems because of your food, they will send a signal to the responsible Gatekeeper. The Gatekeeper will then send you signals (stiff muscles, pain in the joints) in order to fix your food.

The point is there is no point!

How do the Gatekeepers talk to you when they have to warn you:

The neck

The neck is responsible for the organs

    a. on the level of the eyes and above; and

    b. in the back side of the body from above to the neck till the upper back (thoracic vertebra T3); and

    c. in the front side of the body, from the neck including the throat till (but excluding) your manubrium.

When the neck is misused (by limited or excessive movements) during your day, it will start warning you. The first alarm is stiff neck muscles. These will dramatically decrease the flexibility of the neck and restrict its movement. For example, you will not be able to rest your chin on your shoulder without moving the latter, bring your ear close to your shoulder, bring your chin down to touch your chest or bring your head close to your back.

When you do not pay attention to the stiff muscles around your neck joint (atlantoaxia), the neck will send you an alarm downwards, to the next bone (vertebra) of your spine. If you ignore the alarm, the pain will continue and reach your upper back (T1-T3), and then also your throat. Then, you will get a hump in your neck. After all these alarms and signals, the neck will give you pain in the neck joint itself. If you do not fix this pain, your neck will start to affect your organs in the area which belongs to it.

The jaws

The jaws are responsible for the organs:

    a. on the level of the eyes and below (everything in the head that the neck is not responsible for);

    b. the area around the front line of the body (nose, chin, throat, middle of the chest till the diaphragm).

When you use your jaw in a very limited way, the muscles around your jaws will start to get stiff (and this includes all the muscles in the jaws' area of responsibility). Eventually, you will not be able to open your mouth enough to put your wrist vertically inside your mouth (this is the minimum level). After this alarm, the jaw will start to affect your organs in the area that belongs to them.

The shoulders

The shoulders are responsible for the organs:

> a. In the back part of the upper body from thoracic vertebra T3 downwards till T12;
>
> b. In the front part of the upper body from shoulders downwards until the diaphragm (excluding the jaws' area of responsibility);
>
> c. arms including elbows, hands, and fingers.

When you do not circle your shoulders and move them in all directions more than you have to, the shoulder will start alarming you by making your shoulder muscles stiff. If you do not pay attention to these stiff muscles, the shoulder will send you an alarm to the elbow. And if you do not fix this problem, your shoulder will send an alarm to your wrist. If you continue ignoring this, your shoulder will send the pain to your fingers (your fingers will also get curved). After all this, you will be warned one last time by the pain in the shoulder itself. After all these alarms and signals, the shoulder will start to affect the organs in the area which belongs to your shoulder.

The hips

The hip is responsible for the organs of the body from diaphragm downwards. This includes lower back (5 lumbar vertebrae) and the last part of the spinal column (sacral curve: 5 vertebrae of sacrum and 4 vertebrae of coccyx); this also includes the legs all the way down to your toes.

When you do not circle your hips and move them in all directions more than you have to during your day, the hip will alarm you by stiff hip muscles. If you do not pay attention to the stiff muscles, the hip will send an alarm to your knee. And if you do not fix this problem, your hip will send an alarm to your ankles. If you continue ignoring this, your hip will send an alarm to your toes: The toes will start getting curved; they will be too close to each other or will get under each other. After all those signals, you will be warned one last time by the pain in the hip itself. If you do not take any action, the hip will start to affect the organs in the area which belongs to your hip.

Start to move your Gatekeepers more than you have to during your entire day in all directions, in order to fix the damage and not to get the same or other problem again.

Doing Zero Technique when you do not have any damage is as important as when you have it. In other words, preventing health problems is always better than treating them!

How was your day tomorrow?!

To understand Senda Zero Technique for fixing a damage in your body, imagine you have a river and there is a big stone stopping the flow of the river from the Roads to the Castle. Your mission now is to remove that stone by giving more force to the water flow. You remove this stone by working on the Roads or, in case they are not available, directly on the Gatekeepers (e.g., the jaw joints do not have Roads).

What you have to know before using Zero Technique

The jaw joint is a Gatekeeper and a road at the same time. The feet and hands have no control over the jaws.

The Roads in the body have the following areas of responsibility:

- The feet (ankles and toes) are responsible for the bones, joints and organs in the whole body (except the jaws).

- The hands (wrists and fingers) are responsible for the muscles, nerves and organs in the whole body (except the jaws).

- The jaws are responsible for the bones, joints, muscles, nerves and organs in the jaw area (as explained above).

Feet

The feet can be used to fix the damage to the joints, bones or organs in your body.

1- The big toe controls the area of the responsibility of the neck as described in subsection "The neck".

2- The index toe (the one beside the big toe) controls the lower back till the hips (5 vertebrae of the lumbar curve) and the organs on the corresponding level.

3- The middle toe controls the hip, the last parts of the spinal column (9 vertebrae of the sacral curve) till the knee and the organs on the corresponding level of the body.

4- The ring (fourth) toe is for the part of the legs from the knees till the ankles and for the part of the hands from the elbows till the wrists.

5- The small toe is for the area of responsibility of the shoulders as described in subsection "The shoulders", excluding the part from the elbows to the fingers.

6- The ankle is for the ankle and the wrist. The ankle is also responsible to keep the channels clean.

Hands

The hands can be used to fix the damage to the muscles, nerves or organs in your body. The control areas of the fingers correspond to the control areas of the toes as follows.

1- The thumb controls the same area as the big toe.

2- The index finger controls the same area as the index toe.

3- The middle finger controls the same area as the middle toe.

4- The ring finger controls the same area as the ring toe.

5- The small finger controls the same area as the small toe.

6- The wrist is for the wrist and the ankle. The wrist is also responsible to keep the channels clean.

The notation used in the map below is the following.

N = Neck   L = lower back

H = Hip   E/K = Elbow and knee

S = Shoulder   A = Ankle   W = Wrist

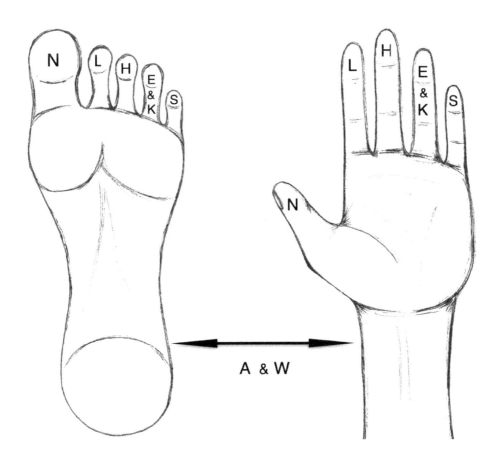

Zero Technique

Follow the steps described below when you have problems with your joints.

1- Use your hand to pull slowly the problematic toe straight backwards (Flex) towards your body till your maximum; the pain will stop you from pulling your toe even more backwards. Hold for a few seconds.

2- Keep your toe straight and pulled backward, then start to bring your toe to the left. Look for the point of pain; if you do not find it, bring your toe to the right till you reach the point of pain. When you find the pain, hold for a few seconds.

3- While keeping your toe straight – pulled backward and brought to the left or to the right – start rotating your toe left and right till you get to the next point of pain. Hold for a few seconds.

4- Release your toe; actively close your toes into a "fist" and keep it for a few seconds.

5- Move each bone of the toe separately in all possible directions till you reach the point of pain. Hold there for a few seconds.

6- Pull the same toe out of its joint (Lisfranc's joint[19]) slowly and keep it straight. Repeat the 4 steps above slowly while keeping your toe pulled out.

7- Move the foot of the toe you have just worked on in all possible directions. Look for the point of pain in your ankle while moving your foot around. Hold for a few seconds in each point of pain.

After completing these steps, start working on the Gatekeeper of the damaged or problematic part by actively moving this Gatekeeper in all directions more than you have to.

If you have pain in your joints, use the toe on the same side of your body. If it is the left knee, work on the left ring (fourth) toe. If it is the left shoulder, work on the left small toe. If it is the left hip, work on the left middle toe. If it is the lower back, work on the left and right index (second) toes. If it is the neck, work on the left and right big toes.

---

[19] If you follow these steps to work on your fingers, this would be MCP join.

1- Use your hand to pull slowly the problematic toe straight backwards (Flex) towards your body till your maximum

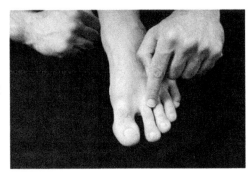
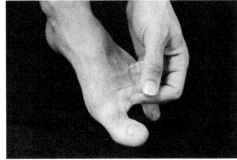

2- Keep your toe straight and pulled backward, then start to bring your toe to the left... right

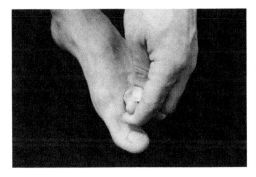
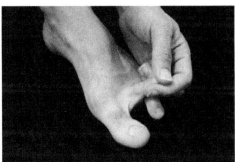

3- While keeping your toe backward start rotating your toe left and right

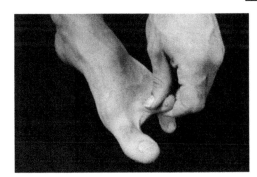
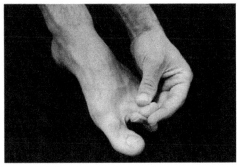

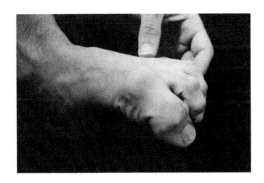

4- Release your toe; actively close your toes into a "fist" and keep it for a few seconds.

5- Move each bone of the toe separately in all possible directions till you reach the point of pain.

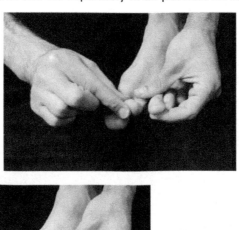
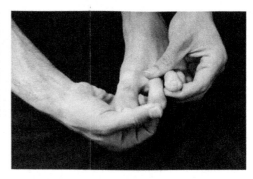

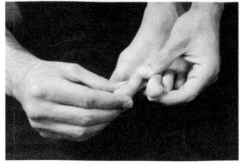
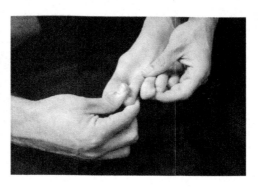

6- Pull the same toe out of its joint (Lisfranc's joint) slowly and keep it straight. Repeat the 4 steps above slowly while keeping your toe pulled out

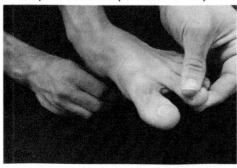
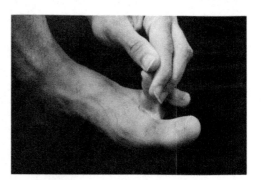

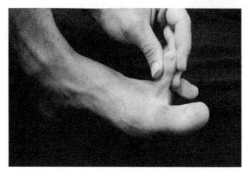
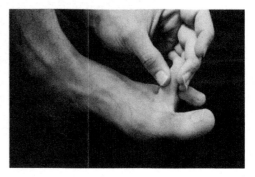

7- Move the foot of the toe you have just worked on in all possible directions. Look for the point of pain in your ankle while moving your foot around. Hold for a few seconds in each point of pain.

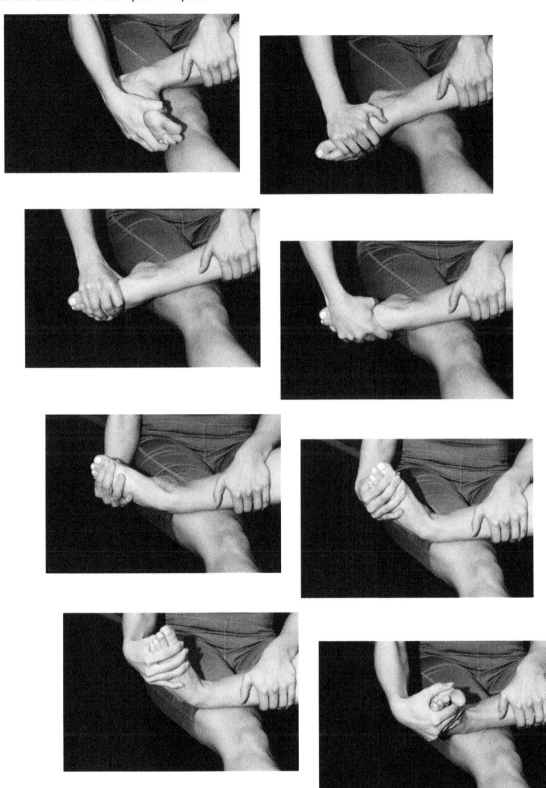

Muscle problems

When the problem is with your muscles, follow the same steps of the Zero Technique for your fingers and wrists instead of toes and ankles.

If you have pain in your muscles, use the finger on the same side of your body. If it is the right knee, work on the right ring finger. If it is the right shoulder, work on the right small finger. If it is the right hip, work on the right middle finger. If it is the right part of your lower back, work on the right index finger. If it is the right part of your neck, work on the right thumb.

1- Use your hand to pull slowly the problematic finger straight backwards (Flex) towards your body till your maximum

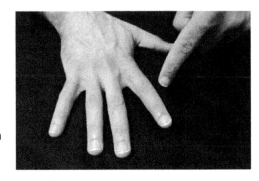

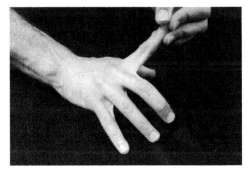

2- Keep your finger straight and pulled backward, then start to bring your finger to the left... right till you reach the point of pain.

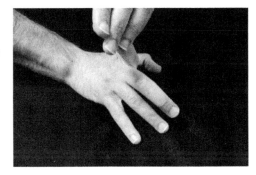

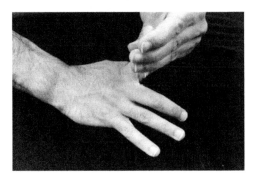

3- While keeping your finger straight - pulled backward start rotating your finger left and right

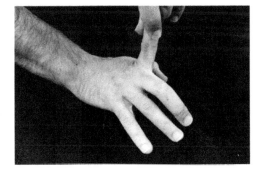

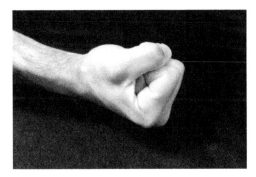

4- Release your finger; actively close your hand into a "fist" and keep it for a few seconds.

5- Move each bone of the finger separately in all possible directions till you reach the point of pain.

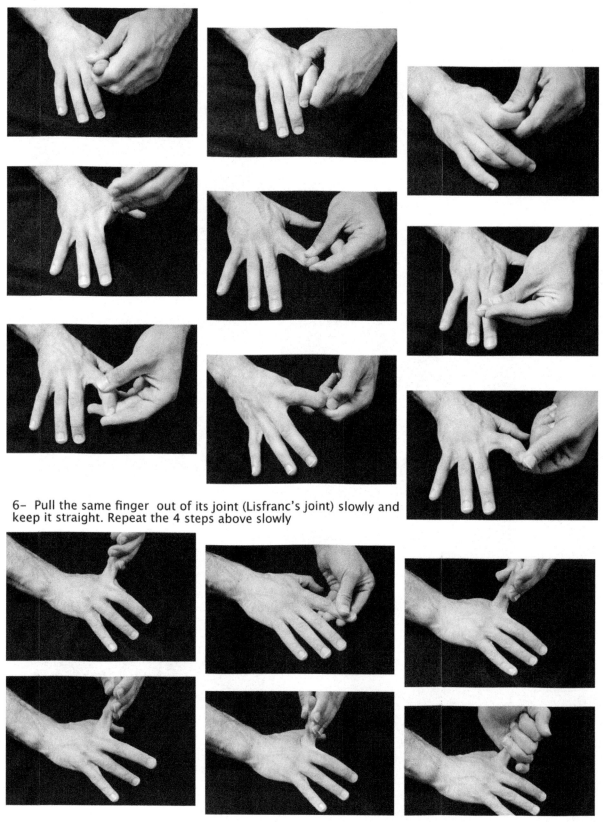

6- Pull the same finger out of its joint (Lisfranc's joint) slowly and keep it straight. Repeat the 4 steps above slowly

7-   Move the hand of the finger you have just worked on in all possible directions. Look for the point of pain in your wrist while moving your foot around. Hold for a few seconds in each point of pain.

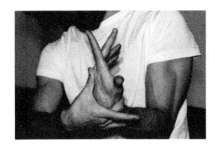
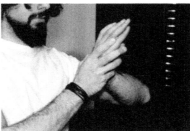
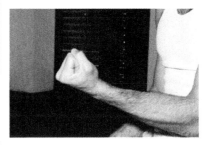
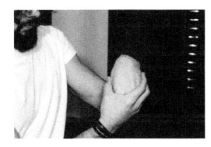
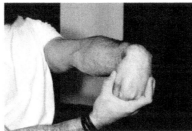
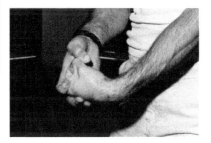
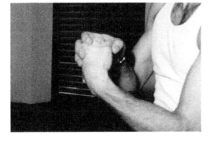
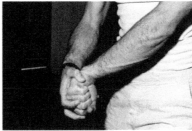
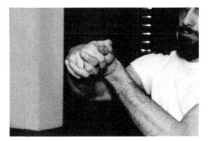
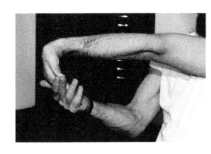
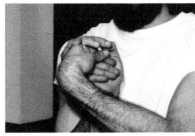

Stop wasting your chance to be a legend

When the problem is in the bones or the nerves, it will help you to work on the closest neglected gatekeeper. For the jaws, that would probably be the neck or the shoulders. If the problem in the neglected gatekeeper is not old or huge, move this gatekeeper in all possible direction. If the problem is huge or old, follow Zero Technique (toes/fingers for bones/nerves).

When you have a problem with your nerves or bones, cross your fingers or toes. To know which fingers/toes you have to cross, consider the following.

Nerves

For the nerves, bring the finger corresponding to a Gatekeeper over its neighbor finger and pull these fingers backwards. Then follow the steps of the Zero Technique for fingers and wrists.

Examples for the pain caused by a pinched nerve.

1- The pain is felt from the right elbow downwards till the right forearm or wrist. Work on the right hand, cross the small finger over the ring finger.

2- The pain is felt in the left lower back. Work on the left hand, cross the middle finger over the index finger.

3- The pain is in the Gatekeeper nerve only. Work on the corresponding finger only.

4- The pain is in the left middle and left ring fingers. Work on the right hand and cross the right middle finger over the right ring finger.

5- You are missing your right hand. The pain is in the right big toe. Work on the left hand and cross the left middle finger over the left ring finger.

6- The pain is in both knees or feet, for example, in big and index toes. Work on the left and right hands, cross the middle finger over the ring finger.

7- The pain is felt from the neck to the left arm. Work on the left hand: pull the thumb and the small finger (Loney) at the same time. You must not cross a Gatekeeper finger with another Gatekeeper finger, but you can pull both of them backwards at the same time.

8- The pain is in the left eye, e.g., from migraine. Work on the left small finger and left thumb.

9- The pain is in both hands (wrists and fingers). Work on the Gatekeeper. Move the shoulders in all possible directions. It will help to also work on the small toes and ankles (yes, on your feet).

1– The pain is felt from the right elbow downwards till the right forearm or wrist. Work on the right hand, cross the small finger over the ring finger.

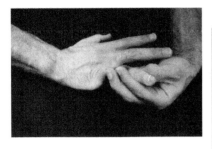 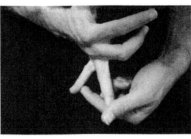 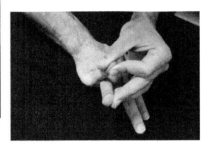

2– The pain is felt in the left lower back. Work on the left hand, cross the middle finger over the index finger.

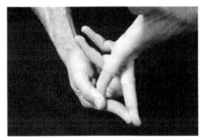 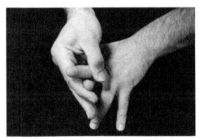

3– The pain is in the Gatekeeper nerve only. Work on the corresponding finger only.

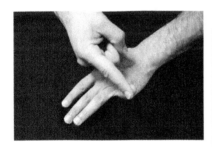 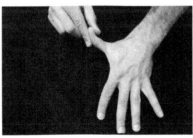 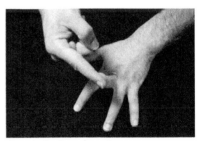

4– The pain is in the left middle and left ring fingers. Work on the right hand and cross the right middle finger over the right ring finger.

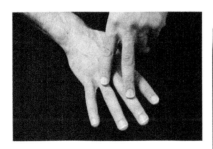 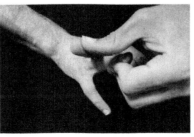 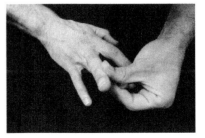

5-   You are missing your right hand. The pain is in the right big toe. Work on the left hand and cross the left middle finger over the left ring finger.

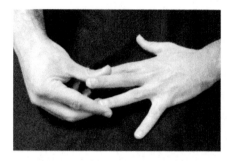
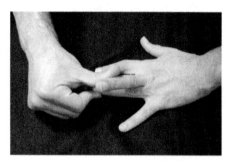

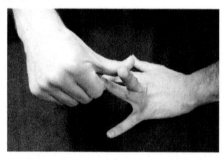

6-   The pain is in both knees or feet, for example, in big and index toes. Work on the left and right hands, cross the middle finger over the ring finger.

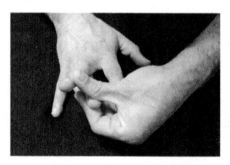
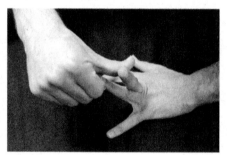

7-   The pain is felt from the neck to the left arm. Work on the left hand: pull the thumb and the small finger (Loney) at the same time. You must not cross a Gatekeeper finger with another Gatekeeper finger, but you can pull both of them backwards at the same time.

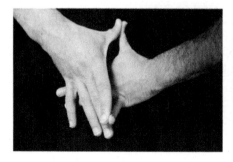
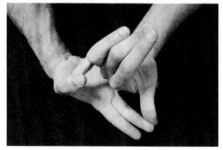

8– The pain is in the left eye, e.g., from migraine. Work on the left small finger and left thumb.

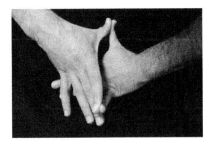 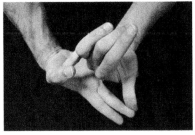

9– The pain is in both hands (wrists and fingers). Work on the Gatekeeper. Move the shoulders in all possible directions. It will help to also work on the small toes and ankles (yes, on your feet).

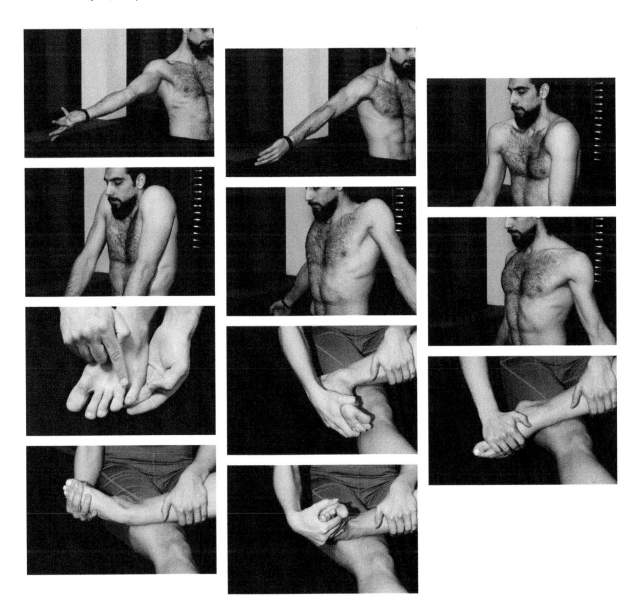

Whenever possible, bring the broken bone back to its place. If you have the gypsum applied, follow the examples below that you can manage. Do it even after the gypsum is removed to let the broken bone heal faster.

Bring the toe corresponding to a Gatekeeper under its neighbor toe and pull these toes backwards. Then follow the steps of the Zero Technique for toes and ankles.

Examples for the pain caused by a broken bone.

1- When a left forearm bone is broken, work on the left foot, cross your small toe under the ring toe.

2- When the left thigh bone (femur) is broken, work on the left foot, cross your middle toe under the ring toe.

3- If the broken bone is in a Gatekeeper joint, work on the toe for the corresponding Gatekeeper (either left or right). The exception is the neck, for which you must work on both left and right big toes. For a jaw break, it will help to work on both big toes. In any event, you must not cross any toes.

4- If the broken bone is in the left foot, left ankle or left big toe, work on the right foot, right ankle or right big toe.

5- In case you are missing your right foot. If the broken bone is in the right hand, right wrist or right middle finger, work on the left foot, left ankle or cross the left small toe under the ring toe. This is because the small toe is the shoulder Gatekeeper toe and is responsible for the fingers.

6- If both hands are broken, work on both feet, cross the small toe under the ring toe.

7- If you break one of the ribs on the right side, work on the right foot: pull the small toe and the middle toe at the same time. This is because the broken rib is between 2 Gatekeepers: right shoulder and right hip. You must not cross a Gatekeeper toe with another Gatekeeper, but you can pull both toes backwards at the same time.

8- If both feet are broken, work on the Gatekeeper. Move the hips in all possible directions. It will help to also work on the middle fingers and wrists (yes, on your hands).

9- In case you are missing your both feet. If both hands are broken, work on the shoulder Gatekeepers. Move the shoulders in all possible directions.

1– When a left forearm bone is broken, work on the left foot, cross your small toe under the ring toe.

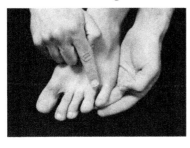 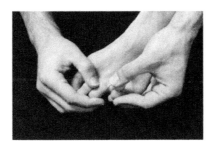 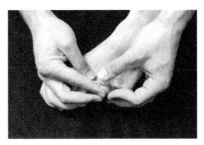

2– When the left thigh bone (femur) is broken, work on the left foot, cross your middle toe under the ring toe.

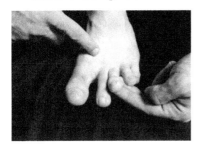 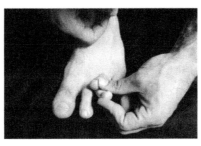 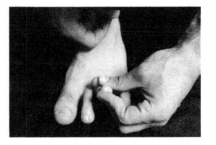

6– If both hands are broken, work on both feet, cross the small toe under the ring toe.

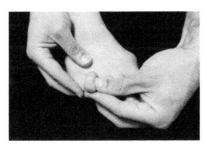 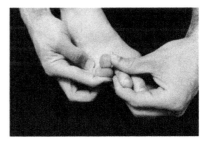

7– If you break one of the ribs on the right side, work on the right foot: pull the small toe and the middle toe at the same time.

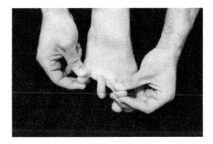 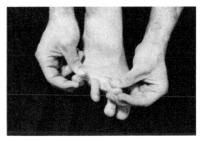

After finding out which two fingers/toes you have to cross or pull, keep them straight while pulling backwards towards your body. Hold for a while. Then do the 7 steps of Zero Technique for each finger/toe of the two fingers/toes you just worked on (cross or not crossed). If the pain in the nerve did not get better, push the fingers more backwards, then repeat the process again. Be patient if the problem is old or huge.

After doing all the steps (if it was possible), start working on the Gatekeeper of the corresponding part, by moving the Gatekeeper in all possible directions considering the joint movement (not your possible directions) till it gets flexible.

I recommend you to work on the problem step by step and not to try solving it at once. Start from the Gatekeeper joint if the injury/problem is fresh; finish the work with the part of your body that started giving you pain last. Start from this last part if the injury/problem is old; finish by working on the corresponding Gatekeeper.

Shoulders:

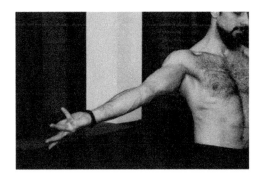 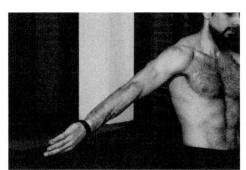

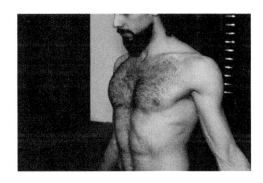 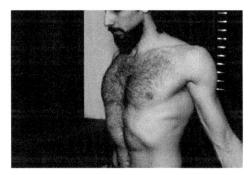

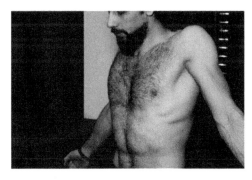 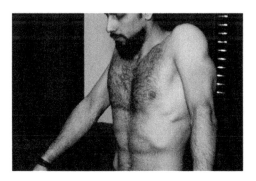

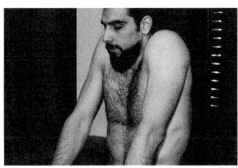 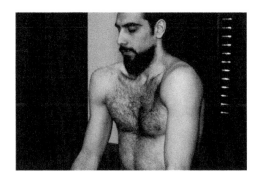

Neck:

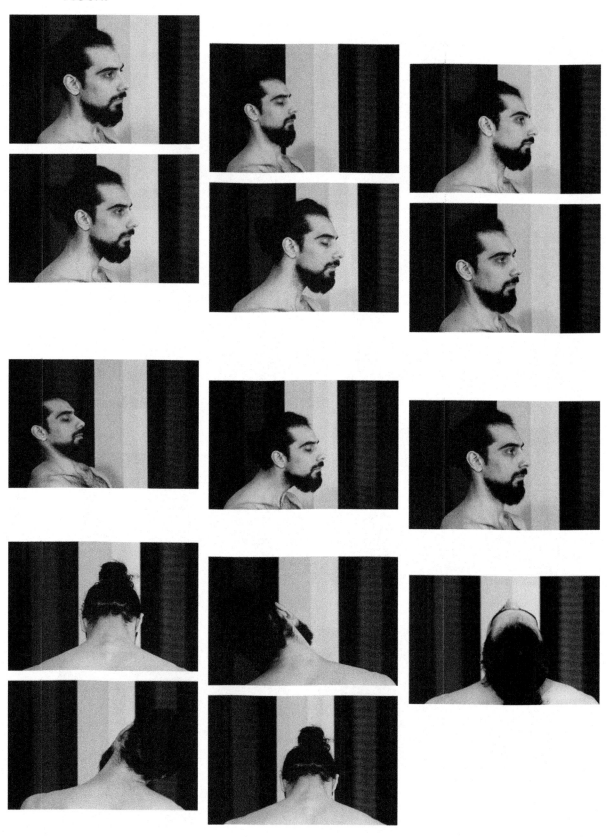

225

Hips

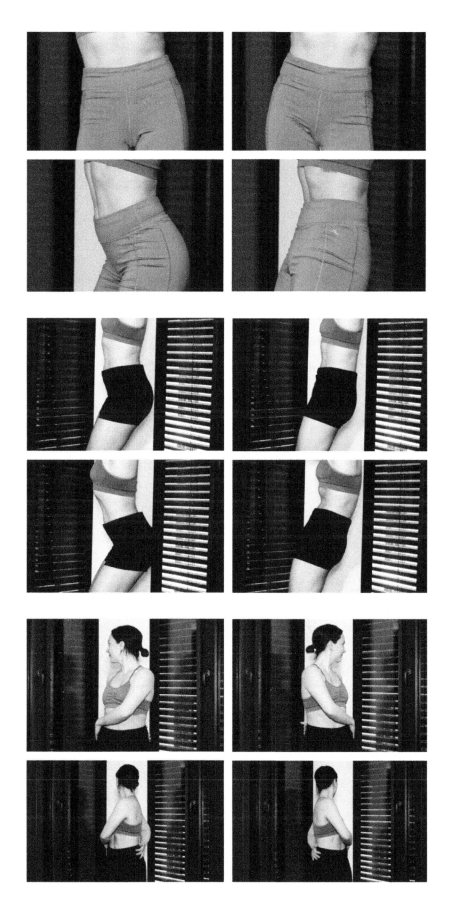

226

To work on muscles, nerves, joints or bones in the jaws, follow the steps described below:

1. Open your mouth to the maximum, then start moving the lower jaw to the left and to the right slowly till you find the point of pain. Hold for a few seconds.

2. Keep your lower jaw on the left or right side at the point of pain, then start moving your lower jaw slowly up and down. Repeat that movement at least 9 times.

3. Make circles of highest possible size with your lower jaw: from the left, go up, then to the right and, finally, down. Repeat the circle at least 5 times. Then make a circle in the reverse direction. Repeat it at least 7 times.

4. Put your tongue out to the maximum. Circle your tongue and move it to all directions. Use the directions and the number of repetitions as described in point 3 above.

To reach better results in fixing your problem, do the following versions of the above:

1. Find your point of pain by moving your head in all possible directions. Once you find that point, do steps 1-4 above.

2. Use your hand as a support to move your lower jaw in all directions.

3. Use your wrist vertically inside your mouth and do the steps 1-3 again.

4. Use your fingers to push the jaws from inside to outside while keeping your mouth opened.

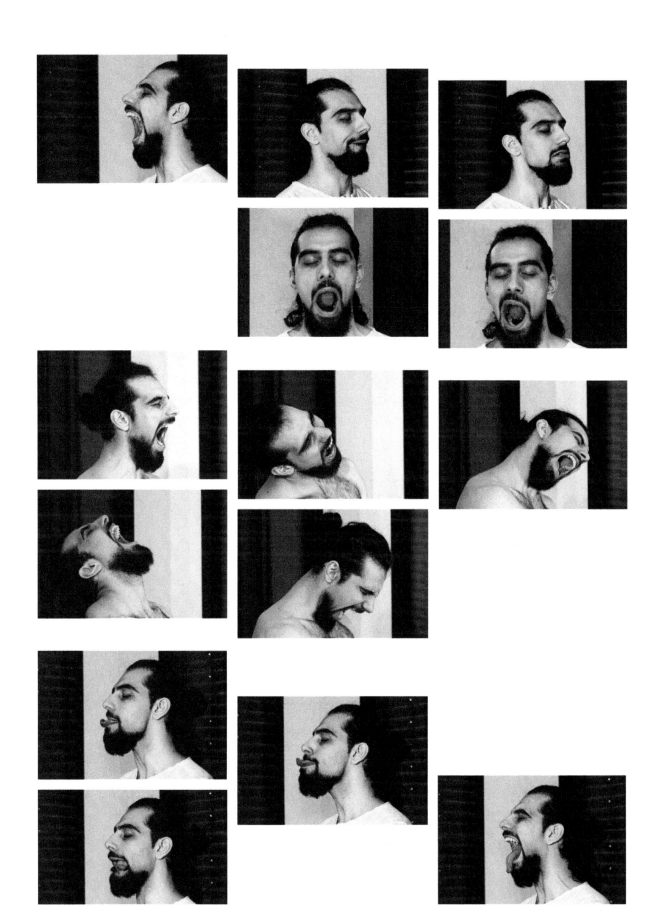

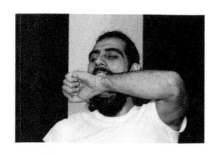

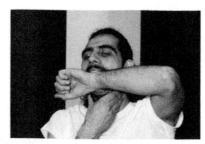

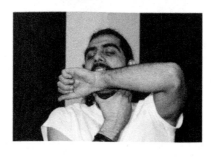

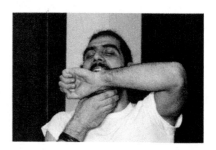

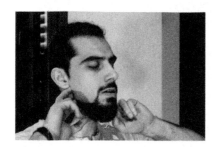

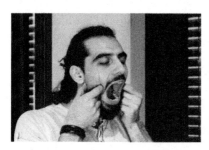

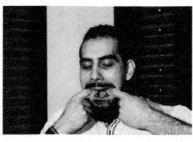

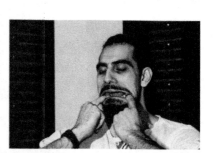

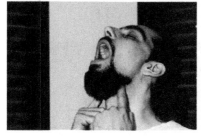

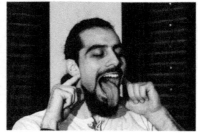

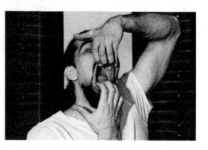

Move your roads while you are awake as explained in Zero Technique, adjusting it to your lifestyle movements (daily routines, job, sport). For example:

1- Move your jaws and tongue in all possible directions before and after eating or drinking.

2- Move your roads before sleeping and after waking up.

3- Move your toes and ankles before leaving home and after coming back.

4- Move your fingers and wrists before and after doing a heavy activity, like writing, typing or cleaning.

5- Move your middle and index fingers from time to time while sitting.

6- Move your roads before starting and after finishing your sport activity. Move the toe or finger responsible for the part of your body that is used in your training.

7- Move the gatekeeper that you are using in your daily routine: move it in all possible directions before, during (if possible) and after the movement.

You will feel the improvement in flexibility, ease and fluency with which your body makes movements after following this technique.

Check your toes and fingers: if one of them is askew, you should be working on it the way explained above till it gets straight. Do that even if you have no pain in your fingers or toes yet. Obviously, if a part of your body does not have a problem, your finger or toe will not be askew to show that problem, unless it is askew because of its broken bone, surgery or inborn feature.

Check your ankles and wrists: if they are not flexible, start to work on getting them flexible. Use the techniques explained above and add your own ways in order to let them move smoothly in all directions. Obviously, if the channels do not have a problem, the ankles/wrists would not be stiff, unless they are limited because of their broken bones, surgery or inborn feature.

Check your gatekeepers: if they are not flexible, start to work on getting them flexible by moving them smoothly in all directions.

You know the details – you are confused, you do not know the details – you are lost. The solution is to go from the end (result) all the way to the beginning (root).

Conclusion

All the techniques presented in this book are just basics. You should build them into your day and add other techniques to make them your own. Your own technique will fit the body you are living in.

If you have a problem in any of your joints or bones, work on the feet. If the problem is in any of your muscles or nerves, work on the hands.

If the problem is in the jaws, it can only be released by working on the jaws. It helps the problem in the jaws a bit to work on the hands or feet as explained above.

After working on your roads (jaws, feet, and hands), start moving the gatekeeper that is neglected or damaged. Move that gatekeeper in all directions more than you have to.

Imagine your body system is a pyramid: the top is a gatekeeper, the middle is the hands, and the base is the feet. Always work from bottom to the top of this pyramid: start with the toes, then work on the fingers and finish with the gatekeeper. If you do not follow this way, you will damage the problematic part of your body further. Never end the process with the toes after working on the fingers.

Life is unfair when you go behind it and life is fair when you ignore it.

Credentials

Author: Emeel Safie, BA.

Editors: Dr. Vilen Lipatov and Emeel Safie, BA

Photography: Emeel Safie, supported by Friederike Hebeler, Süreyya Safie.

Design: Emeel Safie.

Models: Friederike Hebeler, Süreyya and Emeel Safie.

Drawing: Friederike Hebeler.

Acknowledgements

I am grateful to Dr. rer. nat. Jonas Hellhund, Friederike Hebeler, LLM, Süreyya Safie, BA, David Tran, BSc, Thomas Lang, BA, for their comments and suggestions, and Piera Schmincke for her photo editing advices.

I want to thank everyone who supports and believes in Senda, especially my Parents Mohammad Safie and Nahla Yones; my Wife Süreyya Safie; my Brother Alexander F. Müller; my family team at Senda movely livly UG Company Friederike Hebeler and Süreyya Safie.

Special thanks to Josip Dalic, MA, and Dennis Sahin, BSc, for believing in Senda and allowing me to start sharing its techniques in their Personal Training Studio in Frankfurt am Main, Germany. I am also grateful to them for being able to use the Studio for taking pictures included in this book.

Please visit our website www.sendamove.com for translations and any future collaboration.

Printed in Great Britain
by Amazon